Natural Hormone Health

Natural Hormone Health

Drug-free ways to manage your life

Arabella Melville

THORSONS PUBLISHING GROUP

First published 1990

British Library Cataloguing in Publication Data
Melville, Arabella
  Natural hormone health.
  1. Medicine. Natural remedies
  I. Title
  615.535

  ISBN 0-7225-1956-7

Published by Thorsons Publishers Limited, Wellingborough,
Northamptonshire NN8 2RQ England

Typeset by Burns & Smith Ltd, Derby

Printed in Great Britain by Mackays of Chatham, Kent.

10 9 8 7 6 5 4 3 2 1

Contents

To Annabel, Clarissa, Jumper and Spot-Ear

Acknowledgements

Books develop over years of thinking, talking and reading. This one grew from my own experience of hormone difficulties, and the need to overcome them through understanding, and I cannot remember or fully acknowledge all the people who have helped me in my personal search for knowledge. All I can do is offer my thanks to a few individuals who have freely shared their knowledge and intuitions with me.

My partner, Colin Johnson, has stimulated my thinking and helped through frequent discussions and valuable comments on the first draft of the book. I have learnt more from Colin than I can ever hope to say.

My friends Chris and Sally Parsons have contributed over many years to my understanding, particularly of the technical details of nutrition. I thank them both from the bottom of my heart.

A variety of experts and organizations have freely contributed to my research efforts. I am grateful to Belinda Barnes of Foresight, Kate Hunt of the MRC Medical Sociology Unit, Glasgow, Derek Bryce-Smith of Reading University, the Women's Health and Reproductive Rights Information Centre, Women and Medical Practice, Maryon and Alan Stewart of the Women's Nutritional Advisory Service, Stephen Wright and Malcolm Whitehead.

Finally, I should like to thank the people who have encouraged me in my work – my mother, Joan Melville; my agent, David Grossman, and Rosemary Kingsland, whose enthusiasm set me back on course when I was losing heart.

Introduction

I have yet to meet a woman who has never had hormone problems. Problems with periods, pre-menstrual tension, menopause and fertility are an almost universal experience in developed countries and they are getting more severe. Hormone treatment of all kinds is growing steadily more popular, as are drastic surgical operations for hormone-related illness. One effect is the rise in the number of hysterectomies due partly to a phenomenal increase in abnormal uterine bleeding – up 73 per cent between 1971 and 1981.

Yet this need not be so. These problems can be solved by natural means which are both safe and effective, and which offer a better quality of life in the long term. The solutions are not demanding, yet the benefits that can be derived from them are profound.

The deeper I delved into the detailed research that was necessary to write this book, the more I became convinced of the importance of maintaining a healthy hormone balance. Even fit women need to be aware of the action they should take to support their hormone health because imbalance can develop insidiously over years, producing problems that can have dangerous consequences. Long term hormone imbalance shortens life and prevents women from enjoying their day-to-day existence.

It is a strange paradox that the hormones which are fundamental to our female nature also make us prone to so much illness. I believe that women are designed to be strong; after all bearing and rearing children requires great resilence. Yet many women today see themselves as delicate, their bodies unreliable and unpredictable, constantly afflicted by the internal chaos of hormone fluctuations. Something is going wrong with our lives, creating imbalance that damages our health and happiness.

This book explains about the factors that affect our hormones, giving women knowledge and power to make changes in their lives that will allow them to create the best hormone balance. This strategy has been proved effective in the short term and it provides benefits without risk in the long term. By understanding our hormones and their fluctuations, we can free ourselves from disruptive chaos without risking medical or surgical intervention. This is the way to get the best out of life and enjoy the long, healthy and productive life of a well-balanced woman.

To be free of problems with menstruation is a desire shared by all women. We should be able to enjoy our femininity and the key to this lies in understanding our hormones, the most delicately balanced system of our bodies, so that they are not thrown out of kilter by the pressures and apparent conveniences of modern life.

The cost of hormone imbalance is enormous, both to ourselves and society. We may need to spend days in bed, our homes are disrupted by emotional distress, our jobs are affected. The male-dominated business world penalizes affected women while husbands curse and children despair.

Women suffer more ill-health than men and consult doctors more often. But when gynaecological problems are subtracted from total consultation rates, women are less prone to other types of illness; hormone-related illness more than accounts for the extra number of treatments required by women. If our hormones were as stable as are men's, we'd be a lot healthier than they are; but because they're changing and cycling all the time in a relatively uncontrolled manner, women suffer. Many of the serious diseases to which we are subject can be attributed to hormone imbalance, and all our illness is made worse by it.

Many women feel that the only solution is to accept their hormones as a 'problem' and get on with life as best they can. We may be told that we'll be OK if we have babies, or that we've just got to muddle through until we're past menopause. If things get too bad, we'll be offered drug treatment, usually synthetic hormones. And when medicine doesn't solve the problem, there are surgical options, notably hysterectomy. But none of these actually get to the root of the problem, rebalancing our hormones so that life becomes as productive and enjoyable as it should be.

All drug therapy has drawbacks, often major ones. Synthetic hormones can trigger problems that we never previously suffered from, and any hormones we take disrupt our body's natural balance. Balance is very hard to maintain when we add haphazard doses of hormones to an already unbalanced system. Taking anything that increases or decreases the levels of particular hormones in the body is a hit-or-miss process that's liable to produce all sorts of side-effects.

The real answer lies in understanding. When we know what factors naturally influence our hormones, we can consciously adjust our lifestyles to achieve a balance which does not disrupt our everyday lives but maintains our bodies and minds in a state of optimum health.

Every aspect of lifestyle can influence hormone balance, just as hormone balance in turn profoundly influences every aspect of our lives. But modern lifestyle take little or no account of women's special needs. The food we eat, the relentless nature of everyday demands, the chemical pollutants that get into our bodies and the constantly changing structure of many of our lives all affect our hormones and so when our bodies' needs are not completely met, we suffer the ills to which women are prone.

Good nutrition is a crucial determinant of hormone health. But modern farming practices and food processing make it difficult for women to get all the micro-nutrients they need. In addition, our food and environment are increasingly polluted with substances that act as anti-nutrients, adding to the burden on our health. Physical activity is another essential requirement of good health; but how many women know just how active they should be and what sort of exercise they need to protect their bodies? These and other factors which influence hormones are explained in this book.

Natural hormone health means health for the whole woman; glowing health that gives you the energy you need to get the best out of every day, whatever the time of the month, whatever the time of your life. When your hormones are in balance, you will have access to all the strength, power and productivity that is a woman's birthright. At every stage of your life—from growing girl through motherhood to old age—you will be able to enjoy getting the best out of yourself.

Hormones are too important to ignore. You don't need to grit your teeth and put up with the miseries of female problems: they don't have to be problems. This book tells you how to turn your hormone cycles into an asset and tune in to the real power of womanhood.

CHAPTER ONE
Nought But a Jangle of Hormones?

For years, my partner used to have a standing joke about me. According to him, I was either pre-menstrual (two weeks each month), menstrual (one week) or ovulating (two days). He considered I was human for two or three days each month. 'Nought but a jangle of hormones' was his description of me; and despite his chronic exaggeration, it wasn't totally unfair.

I felt it was unfair, of course. I would get very angry that my very real feelings and distress were being dismissed so readily and that he refused to take me seriously, especially when I happened to criticize him. But I had a credibility problem: there was a lot of truth in what he said. In my pre-menstrual days, I *was* irrational; the uncontrollable rage that led me to threaten to murder my adolescent stepson with a sharp kitchen knife *was* underwritten by uncontrolled pre-menstrual tension (PMT); the tiredness and pain that drove me to my bed when my period arrived *was* a symptom of hormone imbalance, and the manic energy that I experienced with ovulation was part of the same hormone roller-coaster.

I remember a similar pattern with my mother: how she would fly into ridiculous tempers, how she would feel persecuted and depressed, how she totally lost her equilibrium when she was going through the hormonal chaos of her menopause. I was an intolerant adolescent then: I had no patience with it all and less comprehension than my own adolescent family showed when they had to cope with my wild swings of mood and energy.

Today, I say proudly (and untruthfully) that I don't have hormones. What I mean is that their ebb and flow is gentle, experienced merely as cyclical change without the pain or misery. I have learned to manage my hormones.

Once, I believed I would only be free of hormone-related

problems when I was an old lady, well past the age of hormonal chaos. In one sense I was too pessimistic: I have not had to wait so long, just long enough to learn the secrets of natural hormone management and to act on my collected knowledge. In another sense I was too optimistic, for my assumption that hormone problems experienced throughout life would leave no residue after menopause was unjustified. Potentially-fatal hormone-related cancers run in my mother's side of the family, alongside all the rest of the implied hormonal chaos. I am well aware that suicide and accidents can make pre-menstrual mental instability fatal. Chronic hormone imbalance can mean you never manage to reach old ladyhood.

My own hormone problems may have been the subject of jokes but in reality, they were no joking matter. If your experience has been anything like mine, you'll know exactly what I mean. Like many women, my problems started at the beginning of adolescence, with my first period. As it becomes established, the menstrual cycle is often irregular and many girls find it difficult to cope with the mess, tiredness, pain, the sheer quantity of blood and its unpredictable arrival. My adolescent years were marred with secret distress from that first day of bleeding which began at such a young age that nobody had thought to warn me about it. I had no ideas what the blood was, where it came from, what I should do; I felt embarrassed because it came from 'down there', a part of my body which made me feel unaccountably ashamed. It was an experience which seared my mind so deeply that it remains totally clear today, thirty years later.

There was a lot of shame to do with menstruation. Shame about the smell, the stains; shame about the source of the blood as I responded to the force of sexual taboos; shame about the whole sordid business. For me, the pain was mainly psychological; it was a decade later in life before I was to experience significant physical pain with my periods.

When other girls in my class began to have periods, I heard about the physical pain some of them suffered; I observed how they would go white and retire to see the school nurse. While I might feel dizzy and black out on the first day of my period, they would be bent double in agony.

Being female began to seem like a cruel affliction.

A decade later, it was my turn to feel the physical pain. It took an IUD (intrauterine device) to stimulate my system into reacting this way; left to itself, my female body had seemed to work quite well after the early years. But I had suffered crippling side-effects with the contraceptive pill and an IUD seemed like a good answer to my contraception problems.

The regular monthly pain brought my periods more sharply into focus but I was prepared to tolerate that because I needed effective contraception. Then I discovered PMT. I say 'discovered' because I had never heard of pre-mentrual problems in 1973, when I realized that I had them. It happened by chance. I was looking back through my diary when I noticed that tear-stained pages occured with remarkable regularity. I found that I suffered cyclical bouts of depression which were at their worst four days before each period. I discovered that I wrote the most irrational things at that time and realized that I could not trust my own judgement.

Pre-menstrual problems vary from woman to woman, and from month to month. I first became aware of psychological symptoms: depression, confusion, anxiety. Later I learnt about physical symptoms such as swelling, breast pain, back, joint and tummy aches. I noticed changes in my diet: normally quite sensible in my eating habits, during the worst of my pre-menstrual days I'd pig out on sweets and chocolate, trying to satisfy sugar cravings. I'd put on weight and my body would get flabby.

Once I had recognized the significance of PMT, I resolved to avoid taking important decisions in the week before my period; all judgements would have to be tentative, to be reconsidered after the first day of bleeding. It's hard to be sufficiently rational to stick to a decision like that when your mind is in pre-menstrual turmoil; and as the years went on and the miseries deepened, I had to take further measures. Rules emerged: no driving when pre-menstrual (accidents would happen then); no interviews; avoid media appearances (what a pity publishers refused to take this seriously!); no impulse buys or sudden changes in the chosen direction of my life. Adjusting to PMT by attempting damage limitation without curing the problem, however, means cutting your life options tremendously.

For me, PMT was only part of the problem. Early books on the subject informed me that a woman would suffer either PMT (caused by one sort of hormone imbalance) or period pain (caused by another). This was not my experience. I had both. Pain and the onset of infection forced me to have my first IUD removed; months later, I tried another, with similar results. By the time I'd finally given up IUDs for ever, severe period pain had become as much a regular and predictable feature of my life as the pre-menstrual syndrome.

With the passing years, the pain worsened. I could no longer attribute it to an IUD, infection, or anything else outside myself, although how far it might have been due to scarring of my reproductive organs as a result of infection, was anyone's guess. Unable to tolerate it any longer, I consulted my doctor. He diagnosed fibroids: small, early ones, but worrying nonetheless. What could be done? A hysterectomy would be the surgeon's answer, he told me. His advice was to ignore the pain for as long as I could.

I decided to find out if I could solve the problem myself. Having done research in medical sociology, I had read about the growing controversy about hysterectomy in the United States and was convinced that this was an operation to be avoided if at all possible. Subsequent research as a health writer taught me that fibroids were hormone-dependent and usually progressive and I began to suspect that I could and should take action to prevent this progression. In addition, I could not help but be aware that my pre-menstrual problems were worse than they had ever been. I suffered migraines, lumpy, painful breasts, aches, a sore and distended belly, tremendous anxiety and depression (nameless dread, we called it), food cravings... I could go on and on. PMT is a many-featured misery.

With all this to contend with, it's no wonder that women like me have been seen as sickly, unreasonable neurotics. That's how I regarded my poor mother when she was disturbed. From the comfort of my current standpoint, I can quite understand why some men will not take women seriously: when your hormones are in chaos, you are not in control of your life. I was, frankly, a mess. And I know there are many others who suffer now just as I used to suffer. I had come to a definite conclusion. It was time I sorted out my hormones.

First I had to understand what I was dealing with. What was the real nature of the problem? What are these powerful hormones whose fluctuations can induce such many-faceted horrors? How do they come to affect so many aspects of our lives, our very selves?

Hormones are chemicals that make things happen in the body. They co-ordinate the biochemical activity that goes on in all our cells, all the time. While the genes we're born with provide the basic blueprint, hormones create the day-to-day changes that determine what actually happens within our body systems.

Produced by organs as diverse as specialized glands such as the ovaries and adrenal glands, to ordinary fat cells, hormones are of many types. They circulate around the body in the blood, continually bathing our tissues. Our cells contain receptors which are sensitive to particular hormones to which they then react; the larger the quantities of hormones or the more sensitive the receptors, the more intense the reactions.

The hormones which concern us here are collectively known as the sex hormones. As a schoolgirl I was taught about oestrogen and progesterone: it is now known that these major hormones form part of an overall pattern that includes a whole variety of other substances. Endocrinologists believe that there are many hormones yet to be discovered, and that related substances which are not recognized as sex hormones interact with them to modify their effects.

Hormones act as the body's chemical messengers, orchestrating our metabolic processes by stimulating changes in body cells. You can visualize them as musical instruments which can play together in harmony, producing a lovely symphony. If they're out of balance, the music is distorted, discordant. You can either decide to take the role of conductor, ensuring that you get harmony, or else let random influences control your hormones and risk cacophony.

Hormones can instruct cells to react to a particular substance, as insulin causes cells to take up sugar from the blood; or to increase their rate of turnover, as adrenalin increases the rate at which we burn fat; or change the internal biochemistry of cells so that they puff up with water or change their shape. In fact, hormones can make cells do just about anything those cells are capable of doing.

Hormone-influenced changes take place throughout the body and brain because hormones circulate everywhere. That's why you'll notice the physical effects of hormone changes at the same time as mental effects. Each hormone may have a variety of effects, depending on the nature and capabilities of the cells on which it is acting. Thus adrenalin, in addition to stimulating fat metabolism, makes your heart pump faster, constricts blood vessels, makes you tense and sharpens your senses. Similarly, sex hormones affect your body function from head to foot—literally! As their levels fluctuate, your mood changes, your body composition changes, and your potential for different types of activity and your overall sensitivity changes. These fluctuating levels vary from woman to woman and they also vary as we grow older.

The body's hormone system is a highly complex and sophisticated one, but, as so often happens in our technological culture, it has been treated as though it were much simpler than it actually is. Western science is built on reductionism, an approach to nature that attempts to look at its parts in isolation to find simple answers. So doctors and scientists have discovered major sex hormones which occur in relatively large quantities— particularly oestrogen, progesterone and testosterone—and they have tried to understand and solve our problems by tinkering with these in isolation.

Fashion and obsession with the latest discovery has led to an over-emphasis on individual hormones. Often this emphasis is governed in large part by the pharmaceutical industry, which profits by selling whatever products it may have developed as a result of these discoveries. Regrettably, this industry funds most of the research carried out by scientists and doctors into new drugs and new treatments.

While commercial issues have a tremendous influence on the direction of research, individual obsession leads some doctors to give undue emphasis to limited aspects of the total hormone picture. Fashion, too, as has been said, plays a part; one hormone may be the cure-all in one decade, another in the next. This is a feature of medical progress of which many lay people are unaware.

One school of thought, led by the well-known gynaecologist Dr Katherina Dalton, seems to regard progesterone as the female hormone of paramount importance. Dr Dalton treats a whole variety of problems with progesterone; and while supplementary progesterone may be helpful for some women, such single-hormone therapy is at best unbalanced and incomplete. Other doctors have emphasized oestrogen and millions of women have been treated with oestrogen supplements. This is now frowned upon by the medical establishment since it was discovered that oestrogen on its own increased the risk of some cancers. Today, mixtures of synthetic progesterone and oestrogen are prescribed in an assortment of guises—as hormone replacement therapy (HRT) and as the contraceptive pill.

Any hormone-supplement treatment that involves using one

or two hormones is inevitably an unbalanced approach to a complex problem that is bound to throw the body's delicate regulatory systems out of balance. You cannot increase the amount of one hormone artificially without producing a whole cascade of unpredictable consequences. First, the body will decrease natural production of the extra hormones you take in an effort to return to balance; with some hormones, the body's struggle to overcome the unnatural increase over a long period of time will mean that production of the hormone is permanently inhibited. This may take a long time to detect; with steroid hormones, once widely used for allergies and arthritis, the effects can be damaging and irreversible. Long-term damage has now been demonstrated with some of the hormones used in early versions of the contraceptive pill: in some women, suppression of natural hormone production leads to lasting infertility. Nobody can yet be sure of all the effects of long-term treatment with any hormone.

Since the body's hormone systems are all interlinked, we may never know just how administration of a particular hormone will affect an individual. We can be sure, however, that there will be many repercussions. Simple-minded tinkering is frankly dangerous.

Our culture's preference for over-simplification has another effect. Instead of looking at the hormone issue as a whole, doctors and scientists have studied problems in isolation. We have come to treat period problems as though they were fundamentally different from the problems of pregnancy, post-pregnancy, and menopause; we behave as though imbalance in one situation doesn't relate to imbalance in another.

The underlying causes of the widespread pain and misery that accompanies hormone problems are often ignored altogether. Women are offered the quick 'techno-fix': take this for your PMT, that for your pains, the other for your menopausal symptoms. Nobody seems to acknowledge that these are all part of the same big problem: hormone imbalance due to a lifestyle that doesn't meet women's needs. It's a lifelong problem and it's one that we can solve by natural means—without risking damage to our delicate bio-chemical balance.

In order to do this, we need to focus on the primary reasons for hormone imbalance. We need to consider the substances that our bodies need to produce hormones in their proper quantities, and those that allow our body cells to respond properly to them.

We need to know something about the creation and metabolism of hormones within our own bodies. And we need to consider the many forces that can interfere with hormone health.

The answer to hormone-related problems is to take control of all the aspects of lifestyle that affect your hormone systems. This means becoming the mistress of your own life, not a victim of it. It means getting up on to the conductor's rostrum and taking charge of that wonderful orchestra, directing the harmonies of your own personal score.

In practical terms, this involves acting consistently to ensure that you do everything you need to do for a healthy life. You must take responsibility for yourself and shed some responsibility for others if this interferes with your own needs. This may mean being a little more selfish so that you get the rest, exercise, and good food you need. But in the longer term, you will be doing the best thing, not only for yourself, but for all the other people in your life.

Solving hormone problems by dealing with the causes may seem a daunting task but the benefits are marvellous. It means learning about yourself, your deep-seated needs and your individuality. It is a fascinating quest into the very nature of womanhood and one that will produce benefits throughout your life.

When you get your hormone balance right, you will be protecting yourself not just from the regular aggravation of PMT or period pains, and the long haul of menopausal symptoms, but also from all the overspill problems of hormone imbalance such as depression, tiredness and weight gain. You will be reducing your risk of cancer and of heart disease; you will be strengthening your bones and your whole body. And if you plan to have a baby, you will be enhancing the chances of producing a happy, healthy child who will be a delight to you and everyone else.

Woman's hormone problems have been taken less than seriously by the male-dominated scientific and medical establishment. To the degree that they are acknowledged, women have been belittled: we can be excused our foolish behaviour, our anger can be ignored or our changeability glossed over, because we are only female after all, nought but a jangle of hormones. If our whole environment and social structure seems to conspire to make women's lot a miserable one, that's just too bad. If we go crazy at intervals, well, that's in the nature of women: we are known to be irrational. Women have to struggle on throughout, just as our grandmothers did. We are, after all, very resilient creatures.

At last, this sort of acceptance of a position of disadvantage, this willingness to bear pain just because of our sex, is fading. In part, the change reflects the loss of power of the old-testament woman-blaming religions which assert woman's inferior position; in part it reflects the growing strength of women built on feminist thinking and increasing freedom from the demands of child-bearing. Finally, women are asserting their strength, their value in society at large, the importance of female nature and female ways of thinking and perceiving. Our priorities are different from male priorities; and health, both for individuals, for our children and for the planet as a whole, is very high on the list of female concerns.

We cannot express our full potential while we are struggling to cope with damaged metabolic systems. As women, we come into our own when we are both mentally and physically well, when we cannot be dismissed as irrational or unreliable because our hormone fluctuations are out of control. A criminal charge dismissed because a woman has over-reacted during her pre-menstrual phase is a hollow victory; the real victory will be ours when women's insights are valued for themselves, not dismissed. But this requires a precision of balance that we can now achieve only through deliberate action. We cannot afford to be passive victims.

Women like me, whose hormones are inclined to go out of balance and cause problems, can learn to identify and anticipate changing body states and respond appropriately. Our needs change as our cycles fluctuate: to be in control, we have to tune in to what's going on and known what action to take. Your experience is the truest guide you can have; what this book will do is teach you how to respond to the messages you receive from your mind and body.

So stop the jangle—get into harmony!

CHAPTER TWO
Hormone Problems – Why so Common?

When the vast majority of women have hormone-related problems for much of their lives, there must be something very wrong with us—or with our lifestyle. Has Nature made a dreadful mistake, equipping us with systems that go so readily and so drastically out of control? Is this an inescapable reality of women's lives? I do not believe so. I am convinced that hormone problems are normal in our culture in the same way as heart disease has become normal (and indeed heart disease kills more than half the population of Britain), and bunions and corns are 'normal' on our feet. Heart disease is avoidable if we make the right choices about our lives, just as bunions are avoidable if we choose the right shoes. Such problems are consequences of the way we live in this culture, and while we may always be vulnerable to them, we need not suffer nearly as much as we do.

Making the right choices for good health is important in order to get the best out of life. Hormone balance is a crucial determinant of the way we feel, both physically and mentally. When our hormones are out of kilter, it can be difficult to cope with even the basic requirements of our lives. Despite the birth of feminism, women are almost always the nurturers, the people who keep families and social groups on an even keel, the people who care. We are expected to be reliable and constant in our actions; yet we are undermined for a disturbingly large proportion of our lives by wild fluctuations of our hormones.

Are we our own worst enemies, betrayed from within by our hormones?

We cannot know for sure whether women have always suffered from hormone problems, but the evidence that is available points to the conclusion that they are now commoner than ever before. Older women friends tell me that PMT did not seem a common problem when they were young but there are simply no statistics that reveal what proportion of women suffered from problems of this type fifty years ago. Such things as periods and PMT tend not to be mentioned either in novels or in most other records. The combination of generalized prejudice against women (who, since Victorian times, at least, have been seen as nervous, sickly and unreliable creatures), a poor diet and restricted lifestyle, all of which could directly damage hormone systems, produce an unavoidably distorted picture.

If it were possible to measure the incidence of PMT, menstrual problems, and severe menopausal symptoms in other cultures, we might then have convincing evidence that could answer these questions. Unfortunately, the taboo that surrounds the whole issue of menstruation means that such information is extremely scarce.

It is not possible to look to any golden age where women lived in some more natural and appropriate way, where their needs were met more perfectly than today, in order to measure the levels of illness they experienced. What anthropological evidence there is too stained with prejudice to be reliable. Anthropologists were usually male and they simply failed to enquire about women's health. And when menstruation is regarded as evil, unclean or dangerous, as it has been by the majority of cultures, it is little wonder that we know virtually nothing of women's experience of the menstrual cycle as a whole.

Period pain has been recognized for centuries but how common it was, nobody knows. It seems that women suffer more in cultures where the disgust or taboo associated with menstruation is strongest but in our culture, where taboos have lost much of their power, period problems are on the increase. Statistics collected by general practitioners reveal a 73 per cent rise in new cases of abnormal uterine bleeding in the single decade between 1971 and 1981. Consultation rates for period problems are rising and gynaecological surgery is more prevalent too.

PMT was first clearly identified in 1931, when a New York doctor reported on 15 women who suffered from pre-menstrual water retention and nervous tension. Other studies of the phenomenon followed. Some included surveys of the frequency with which women suffered from symptoms of PMT; all recorded a smaller proportion of sufferers than that revealed by recent research. This suggests—though it does not prove — that PMT is commoner now than it used to be.

For me, the most convincing argument is evolutionary. I find it impossible to imagine that we should have evolved in such a way that so many women should be so seriously incapacitated by their hormone fluctuations for so much of the time. Could humans have become arguably the most successful species on this planet if half the race were so badly designed? No: the fault is not in the underlying design (except, perhaps, in the delicacy of its balance) but in the way we run our bodies and our lives. This is where the problem lies.

Rapid changes have been taking place in the way we live. Technology has transformed society within the space of a single lifetime. Food has changed with the development of chemical farming and the food processing industries; insidious chemical pollution has become a frightening but omnipresent feature of our world. With the development of the internal combustion engine and the subsequent increase in car ownership, many women would be horrified if they had to walk as much as people, even young children, habitually had to do every day fifty years ago.

Inevitably, these changes affect our bodies. The changing picture of illness over the course of this century reflects the transformation of our society. Instead of hunger, we suffer obesity and heart attacks; instead of fatal infection, we suffer chronic allergies. We have more long-standing disease, less acute and dramatic illness. The rise in these modern types of illness has been especially dramatic over the past 30 years, with accelerating effects in the last couple of decades. While we may be living longer than our grandmothers, we are certainly not healthier.

Hormone imbalance is one aspect of the more general problem of long-standing illness that afflicts so many people today. When, according to the government's General Household Survey, one third of women report such illness, it's inevitable that this represents a great deal of hormone imbalance. Women between the ages of 16 and 44 had 50 percent more long-standing illness in 1983 than they had in 1972; much of this illness is hormone-related.

Just how common are hormone-related problems today? Surveys produce widely differing estimates, depending on what questions are asked, and what group of women is questioned. The answers they produce may not be reliable either, because some women do not recognize that they have hormone problems. Before that day in Montreal when I looked back through my journal, I had no idea that I suffered from PMT and if someone with a clipboard had asked me about my pre-menstrual experience, I'd have blithely assured that person that I suffered no symptoms. And so it is with other women; those who have never kept a diary where they record feelings and symptoms may fail to see the link between their hormone cycles and changing mental and physical state.

Often, questions about health don't have clear-cut answers. I always hesitate when I'm asked how long my periods last. Should I include those last days when there's just the occasional spot or trickle of blood? Or are they just interested in the days when there's a real flow? What counts as pain? Is that sensation of heaviness in the lower belly pain? What we experience depends greatly on how we're feeling generally, what we're doing, and how we expect to feel. When I'm busy and active I may not notice things that would otherwise be interpreted as painful. How often have you noticed cuts or bruises after you've finished an absorbing outdoor job and wondered how they got there?

Of course, more extreme pain, menopausal flushing or others symptoms *will* be picked up in surveys. But these figures, inevitably, do not represent a precise reflection of the real situation.

Nevertheless, the figures we do have are disturbing. They tell us that the vast majority of women are significantly affected by their menstrual cycles. It's likely that no woman ever gets through life without at some time experiencing pain or distress associated with hormone fluctuations.

Menstrual pain—pain experienced during the monthly flow—is also familiar to almost every woman, although its intensity and regularity varies at different periods throughout life. Menstrual cramping is often worst for younger women; by the mid-twenties or after childbirth, it tends to fade away, sometimes returning in a new form in later life.

Sociologists Annette and Graham Scambler studied menstrual problems in a sample of London women between the ages of 16 and 44. The women were invited to rate their experience of symptoms during 'an average period'. Two-thirds (67 per cent) of the women reported at least one distressing symptom during menstruation; 23 per cent suffered strong or acute menstrual pain, while 15 per cent had severe backache. Irritability, fatigue, depression and anxiety were also very common, as were headaches, swelling and weight gain. Together, these symptoms present a picture of generalized menstrual misery which is not necessarily focused on the reproductive organs themselves.

An experience which so many women share must be regarded to some degree as 'normal' but the boundaries of normal are very hard to establish. I shall never forget the doctor who told me, aged 24, that the pain I was suffering from was 'normal'. I *knew* it was not normal for me: I had 13 years of 'normal' periods to judge it by. In fact I had a serious pelvic infection at the time. One of the problems we confront is that while we know that other women also suffer, we can never really know how much they suffer and whether our own particular distress should be ignored or not.

This can lead to serious problems when a woman consults her doctor for excessive bleeding because the doctor may initiate action which will have important repercussions on her later life. When the amount of blood lost by women who considered their periods very heavy has been compared with the quantity lost by women who thought their period loss normal, no difference has been found. Yet excessive bleeding is a common reason for hysterectomy, a drastic surgical operation.

Putting incidence figures on pre-menstrual distress can be even more difficult because the symptoms are not clear-cut. It is currently estimated that three out of four women suffer from PMT. The Scamblers' figure was 73 per cent, while a street survey carried out by the Women's Nutritional Advisory Service produced a figure of 74 per cent. So by these measures, like menstrual distress, pre-menstrual syndrome must be regarded as normal among women in Britain today.

The most common symptoms of PMT are emotional in origin: nervous tension, mood swings, irritability, anxiety and depression. Next come symptoms largely associated with water retention: swelling of extremities, weight gain, abdominal bloating and breast pain. Many women also suffer from headaches, backache and lower abdominal discomfort.

During the week before and, often, during the first few days of the period, women are likely to find that all sorts of health problems become more severe. Allergies tend to worsen; asthma attacks, for example, may cluster around this time. Epileptic seizures become more frequent. Susceptibility to infections ranging from thrush and herpes to colds and 'flu is liable to increase as the body's immune competence falters.

And finally, as if all this were not enough, your looks can go: hair goes greasy or fly-away, spots erupt, bruises appear spontaneously.

No wonder it's called 'the curse'!

Before we can be free of all this, there is the final hormone hurdle: menopause. 90 per cent of women suffer menopausal symptoms to some degree and this is a grim experience for some women. Menopause can combine many facets of PMT—bloating, weight gain, irritability, depression, sore breasts—with special bonuses of its own, notably hot flushes, chills and palpitations, and menstrual irregularity. Although these symptoms are not severe for most women, only about 10 per cent sail through the change of life without any distress. Longer-lasting effects of hormone change can include osteoporosis (brittle bones), leg pain, hair loss or excessive hair growth, vaginal itching and dryness, and other symptoms which fade into the familiar signs of old age.

The other times in a woman's life when natural hormone swings occur are associated with pregnancy. During pregnancy itself, the many changes in the body necessary to sustain and nourish the baby are orchestrated by the same hormones that fluctuate from week to week in those who are not pregnant; with the end of pregnancy—whether it happens prematurely through miscarriage or abortion, or at term when the baby is born— hormone levels fall precipitously, once again producing distressing symptoms for some women. Post-natal depression (the baby blues) is believed to be one consequence. Depression after miscarriage or abortion is almost universal and the loss of the baby is probably only part of the cause; changes in the hormone balance contribute too.

Other types of hormone-related illness are known to be associated with the way we live. Diabetes, for example, caused by a failure in the way the body manufactures or uses the hormone insulin, was once very rare in every culture. After the adoption of Western patterns of diet and lifestyle, it quickly became extremely common among susceptible people. Among the Nauru islanders of the Pacific, who have been selling their potash-rich islands to buy American luxuries from cola to tinned fruit, the incidence of diabetes has risen to over 50 per cent. Even in

Britain, where we seem to have greater resistance to it, diabetes has risen tremendously over the course of this century. Over the past 30 years alone, childhood diabetes has increased six-fold.

Are the hormone-related problems from which so many women suffer similar to the insulin-related disease suffered by the Nauru islanders? The illness may not be as serious but we can be sure it has parallel causes—changes in diet, behaviour, and other aspects of lifestyle which change the body's hormone levels and the way our cells respond to those hormones.

To answer the question of why hormone problems are so common today, we need to know how lifestyle affects our hormone systems. Some clues can be gleaned from the accumulating information about the sort of measures that can correct these problems.

First, there is the issue of nutrition. Hormones, like the rest of our bodies, are created from the food we eat. In order to create all the hormones we need in sufficient quantities, we have to get enough of the nutrients they're actually composed of, and to make the enzymes and other substances that affect the production, metabolism and functioning of our hormones.

The modern diet is very different from the one which evolution designed our bodies to function on. Although the rich countries of the world are not subject to famine, and we may believe that we are eating good food, many women's diets are distorted by a whole range of pressures that affects them both directly and indirectly.

At an individual level, attempts to lose weight or lack of concern about food needs may damage nutritional status; we may starve ourselves deliberately in the hope of getting slim or more casually, because we don't care enough about ourselves or what we eat. At a social level, industrial control over food production and processing has led to a progressive reduction in the nutritional value of food. A junk food diet washed down with the favourite tipples of Western society—coffee, tea, and fizzy drinks—damages all our body systems, including our hormones. Most thinking women try to avoid junk food but even so they may be harmed by some foods that they do not realize can be damaging, and they may not be getting enough of the nutrients their bodies need.

Nutritional measures—choosing the right foods for your body, avoiding those that could be harmful—form a crucial part of the strategy to improve hormone balance. Diet affects all the hormone-related ailments to which we are prone. The Women's Nutritional Advisory Centre in Sussex has taught many women how to eat to free themselves from pre-menstrual problems and their success rate is impressive. Chapters four and five explain how diet influences hormones and how to choose the right diet.

Sometimes it is impossible to get enough of certain essential nutrients to solve hormone problems with dietary changes alone. This can happen when other influences such as pollution or illness increase our need for particular nutrients. Many women benefit from using nutritional supplements but these require careful, balanced use and understanding. Chapters four, ten and eleven will tell you more.

Physical activity interacts with nutrition to change the way our body uses particular nutrients, and the availability of the most crucial nutrients for our hormone systems is influenced by our activity patterns. Understanding your needs for activity and meeting them can produce spectacular benefits in all types of hormone imbalance. Chapter six explains the physical aspects of hormone health.

In our fast, thrusting culture, we may acknowledge the importance of positive action but fail to recognize its equally important balancing partner: rest. Our needs for rest, recuperation, solitude and time for ourselves, vary with the cycling of our hormones. Women have to have the confidence to assert their right to the quiet times they need. Again, understanding is the key to getting the balance right so that you stay on an even keel and your hormone cycle does not throw you off balance. It can be difficult for busy women, especially those who share their home with families, to get the space and time to meet this need. Chapter seven will give you the knowledge to back up your claim to have adequate rest.

All cultures are a complex whole made up of everyday lifestyle variables, woven into a fabric of attitudes, beliefs and assumptions. How we feel depends to a large degree on the way our experience meshes with the attitudes of our culture. There are direct connections between the parts of the brain that deal with thought and emotion, and the master gland, the pituitary, that directs hormone production, so the parts of our culture that affect our thinking and feeling minds will inevitably affect our body cycles too. This is the most subtle area of natural hormone management but one that should never be ignored because it has crucial implications for the way we experience our hormone fluctuations. Chapters seven and twelve, in particular, delve into these mysteries—though these are themes to which we shall return repeatedly.

The complete answer to the hormone problems that are so common in our society involves examining every aspect of our everyday life. Doctors and scientists have tried to produce simple solutions—take these pills, those pessaries, have this implant or that operation—but inevitably, with such a complex problem, these are unsatisfactory solutions. The influences that damage our hormone systems are pernicious, they undermine us in every way. It makes much more sense to deal with the causes of the problem, rather than attempting to suppress the body's reactions while the damage continues.

CHAPTER THREE
A Subtle Balance

Cyclical change characterizes all natural processes. Woman's nature, in its changeability, the ebb and flow of hormones matched by the waxing and waning of desires, feelings, strengths, is part of the larger pattern of moon and tides, birth and death. Lately, the trend of human culture has been to reject and dominate the natural world from which humankind sprang, rejecting these feminine realities of constant change and distorting the balance of the world itself. Our changeability, judged by narrow male values, becomes unreliability, unpredictability, inferiority. And women so much accept these dominant assumptions, that they lose their own innate wisdom, reject and lose themselves, ceasing to understand the cycles of life. As individuals, we lose that subtle balance that allows us to function effectively, becoming prey to a host of female complaints.

Human activities have perpetrated many horrors on the natural world in the name of progress. We, being part of that nature, join in the suffering; our hormone cycles become a curse.

How many women long, as I used to, for the stable hormones of the male? No pre-menstruals, no menstruals, no menopause, no worries about pregnancy. But with femaleness comes something quite beyond the obvious sex differences. It brings a different way of seeing the world that is a product of the different nature of our bodies.

We hang in a balance of many-changing cycles, interwoven and interacting. This balance is vulnerable to change yet because of its very vulnerability, it is also receptive: a balance that can give us a special vision. This is something that is often recognized, though our culture gives it little value. Women's minds, influenced by the constant cycling of our hormones and our roles as mothers and nurturers, have a flexibility and intuitive understanding that we often fail to appreciate and develop.

Some years ago, I found myself looking after a 16-year-old Libyan student. Young for his age, he had devoted many of his few years to the study of the Koran. Every evening, as I cooked supper, he would talk to me about Islam and the code of behaviour by which he was expected to live as a Muslim. His great challenge was to get me to read the Koran, which he explained was Absolutely True.

One evening I asked him why all the Mullahs were men. He replied nervously, fearing I'd laugh at what was no laughing matter. 'Women can't talk about philosophy or religion, because they've only got half a brain.'

Suddenly I realized that in a curious way, I agreed with him; but because the Koran was written from a male point of view, it failed to acknowledge that from where women stand, men have only half a brain too! Men and women have different ways of seeing, areas of their minds that are individual and hidden from the perception of the other sex. And women's changing hormone balance is part of the difference that is in the whole of her body and mind, the expression of the difference between male and female that pervades every cell of our bodies.

What women can gain from the changing state of their selves is breadth of vision, an ability to see things from many viewpoints, an intuitive understanding of the balance of forces which cannot be measured but only felt. Women who are in touch with their nature know they must always consider the unseen, the changing. This gives us a way of thinking that may be called illogical or unscientific; but science depends crucially on what is known, while women and life are frequently shaped by that which is currently unknown.

Male hormones, by contrast, take a linear course, rising in adolescence, levelling out at maturity, falling after middle age. Not for them the constant ebb and flow, the cycles of conception and loss. The experience of life as a fluctuating balancing act is peculiar to women.

Recent knowledge emphasizes the need to respect the balance of life and the necessity of making allowances for those things we can only surmise. This is where intuition, that leap into the unknown, comes into its own. The idea that our scientific endeavour—for all its achievements—has produced answers to everyday problems looks dreadfully hollow when we face the possibility of massive catastrophe caused by global warming, poisoning, and ozone depletion by modern chemicals.

Woman's nature is a microcosm of the nature of life on earth. We are changeable, but we are no less valuable for that; this is something we need to appreciate, accept and understand. Just as the weather is part changeable, part predictable, and we plan our gardening or our venturing out of doors accordingly, so are we ourselves.

Our hormones, in their constantly changing dynamic balance, are like wildflowers in the woods. As I write this, anemones and bluebells are in their prime, bright reminders of springtime and young life. Around them, brown and crumbling, are the disintegrating remnants of last summer's vegetation. Under the dry bracken, still hidden from casual view, summer plants are rising: rosebay willowherb which will paint the hillside pink in midsummer, mauve balsam to follow in August. There is a continual weaving of cycles; the snowdrops, over now, will sleep until next winter while bracken and brambles spring up to dominate the hillside.

In the same way, our hormones rise and fall, creating many different balances as the months and years progress. Some are produced in large quantities like rosebay willowherb, tall and dramatic; others circulate in smaller amounts but, like the wood anemone, they are still important in their contribution to the whole picture of the way we feel at that time. The wood anemone, a small and delicate flower, will seem to disappear totally when the summer plants are grown tall; but because of the timing of the natural cycles of which it forms a part, the anemone dominates today. Similarly, hormones which are produced in even minute concentrations may have a very great effect when the balance of other hormones is right.

So I do not believe it is particularly useful for women interested in the practical reality of their hormone changes to get caught up in the minutiae of fluctuations in progesterone, oestrogens, luteinizing hormone, follicle stimulating hormone, and the rest. Too much attention to partial pictures produces incomplete solutions that ultimately fail. Understanding your hormones means understanding your own experience and your own personal needs.

Hormones form a closely interconnected web where a change in the level of one affects everything else. They act not only on our bodies, producing the physical signs of the menstrual cycle from the nature of the secretions from our vaginas to the unseen changes in the ovaries, but on our minds and moods. Brain hormones control the ease with which particularly types of nerve transmissions happen; changing their levels determines whether we're likely to yawn or bounce with energy, whether we laugh or cry, and even whether we are more likely to remember happy or sad events. And the brain hormones are part of the same pattern, caught up in the same cycles, as the sex hormones that circulate throughout our bodies.

The hormone picture as a whole is controlled by a small gland in the brain called the pituitary. This hangs like a little round bag from the hypothalamus, the part of the brain that controls emotion and appetite. Connected to the hypothalamus, and continually influencing it, are the 'higher' centres of the brain which give us our senses, memory, creativity and thought. So theoretically at least, our hormone cycles could be controlled by the power of pure thought; I shouldn't be at all surprised if some yogis or similar adepts have demonstrated just that sort of sophisticated mind control. Even in our relatively unsophisticated culture, there is plenty of evidence to demonstrate that our minds affect our hormone cycles; and of course, vice-versa, as every woman who has experienced pre-menstrual rage or nameless dread knows well.

The patterns of changes in the levels of four of our sex hormones during the menstrual cycle are shown in the diagram opposite. This shows three peaks at mid-cycle, with oestrogen peaking first, followed by FSH (follicle stimulating hormone) and LH (luteinizing hormone). While there is plentiful evidence that oestrogen and progesterone levels have an important influence on the way we feel, FSH and LH seem to produce their effects on our reproductive systems without directly changing our moods or behaviour—or at least, without any effects that we recognize.

The body's production of sex hormones varies tremendously depending on our age and where we are in our reproductive cycles. The hormones in girls' bodies cause a growth spurt from about the age of 10 which involves a sudden increase in fat deposition. When they reach a critical weight, reflecting the appropriate balance of fat to lean, the ovarian cycle is initiated.

Our ovaries are responsible for producing the largest quantities of sex hormones from menarche (the first period) until the menopause. Many parts of the body react to oestrogen produced by the ovaries; among other effects, it causes fat to accumulate on

Hormone changes which occur during the menstrual cycle

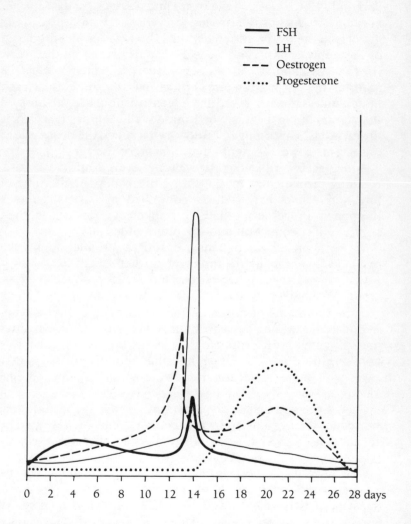

the specifically feminine sites of breasts, hips, buttocks and thighs. The sex organs develop in response to this hormone stimulus, until maturity when they adopt their regular cyclical pattern of fertility and preparation for pregnancy.

The cycle is controlled by the pituitary gland, which produces FSH and LH. Changes in the ovary and uterus stimulate further hormone production. Oestrogen levels rise each month as an egg matures in the ovary, stimulated by LH. Progesterone, produced by the empty egg-sac (known as the corpus luteum) in the ovary, rises after ovulation to support a potential pregnancy; then it falls again as the corpus luteum shrinks towards the end of each month unless the egg is fertilized. Menstruation, the shedding of the uterine lining, begins when these sex hormones reach their lowest levels. This lining re-builds itself through the next cycle to once again create the right environment for the egg.

If the egg is fertilized, progesterone levels continue to rise, reaching their highest levels during pregnancy. At the time of birth—an event that itself is controlled by specialized sex hormones—progesterone falls precipitously. Hormones then control milk production and the return of fertility.

As we approach menopause, oestrogen production by the ovary declines. Finally the time comes when an egg is no longer produced and there is no corpus luteum to produce progesterone. Without progesterone, there's no period; instead there may be symptoms of hormone imbalance. The cycle becomes irregular and eventually ceases altogether; although the ovaries are still active, still producing some sex hormones, their role continues to diminish. Other hormone-producing tissues take over, with more sex hormones being created in the adrenal glands and fat cells, and a new balance ensues.

This always dynamic equilibrium between the different hormones is co-ordinated by regulatory systems orchestrated by the pituitary. It produces constantly changing effects on the body which imply constantly changing needs.

Obviously, if your body is to start producing a high level of any particular substance, all the components needed to make that substance will have to be available. All the enzymes involved in production and metabolism of that substance will have to be there, along with the transport systems that move hormones and nutrients around the body.

If your everyday habits mean that you are barely meeting your needs for the nutrients your body needs to create these enzymes, hormones, or transport systems, then you could be thrown off balance just as your requirements reach their maximum. To maintain the equilibrium of this subtle balance, you need to be sure that your needs are fully met at all times.

As the balance changes with age and pregnancy, your needs change. Other factors—your exposure to toxic stress, the demands of everyday life, your changing body composition—add to the variability as we progress through the years. Every individual is unique; my needs will not be precisely the same as yours, not only because my precise body composition is unique, but also because my biochemistry won't be quite the same as yours. We all have slightly different balances of enzyme systems, slightly different muscle characteristics, slightly different nervous systems and different points of hormone equilibrium. Each person has to get to know herself, tuning into her own body and the way it works best.

This may require a fundamental change in your attitude towards your body. It's an approach based on respect for nature and our own nature; not mind over matter or self-denial, but a genuine acceptance of self. You'll find it easier to achieve a better balance if you can stop condemning, hating or insulting yourself. The difficulties you have had to endure have come about through lack of understanding and the failure to take action based on that understanding, rather than inherent failings. Good health comes not through accidents of fortune, but through choices that we make throughout our lives. Maybe you haven't been making the right choices up to now; probably you didn't know what was right for you.

Understanding your needs comes both from knowledge about lifestyle and how if affects us all, and learning what factors affect you as an individual. Keeping a diary is very helpful; it will give you feedback on the way your hormone fluctuations affect you and the factors which make you feel better or worse. For example, you might note that you regularly feel energetic before your period and desperately tired when it starts. You might find that you can use that energy while avoiding the tiredness by taking heavy physical exercise followed by plenty of sleep just before you expect your period. You may realize that you need more food than usual to fuel the energy without producing a deficit when your hormone cycle moves into its next phase, and your problems get much worse when you neglect to eat regularly.

If you don't work out how to use your energy constructively, you're liable to find it can turn destructive. Staying at home and watching TV could lead you to fret and then, if you live with a friend or partner, to quarrel. When you can anticipate this, you might be able to arrange to go dancing with friends or to book a tennis lesson in advance to ensure that your plans match your changing state as precisely as possible. Once you know how you change from week to week, you may want to tell your partner more about yourself. Your cycles will affect the people closest to you as well as your own life, and alter the nature of your interaction with others.

For example, your sexual tastes are likely to be influenced by your hormone state; breast changes may make you love or hate nipple stimulation, depending on the time of the month. If you get very sensitive pre-menstrually, you may want your sexual partner to leave your breasts alone until your period starts; alternatively, sensitivity may increase the erotic charge of any sex-play that involves your breasts. You may love intense, forceful sex at mid-cycle but prefer it to be slow and gentle at other times; you may feel randy when your period comes and want more sex then. Communication is the key to a more harmonious and satisfying sex life.

Your social desires may also fluctuate with your hormones. Perhaps you like to be alone when your period arrives. Perhaps you enjoy entertaining guests at some points in your cycle, not at others. Take note of these feelings; going against them induces pointless stress.

Any actions you take to achieve a better hormone balance have to be integrated. If you consider only one aspect of your life, for example exercising conscientiously while neglecting rest or diet, you will throw yourself out of balance. If you consider only physical changes without thinking about the way your moods are affected, you may produce internal conflict when your demands on yourself don't take sufficient account of your feelings. Each aspect of life affects every other aspect and we have to acknowledge these links.

We have to be aware, too, that although the effects of our actions may not be obvious in the short term, they can be very important in the long run. For example, if you don't bother with demanding exercise in your thirties, you may not notice any harm at the time. But in due course you will reach your fifties and sixties, when hormone changes can cause bone loss. You will then be more vulnerable to fractures than you need have been.

Had you been active decades earlier (exercise helps keep the bones strong, see Chapter six), you could have reduced the risk.

Sometimes we take deliberate action to try to improve our health, only to find that nothing seems to change. We begin to wonder if it's worth the bother. Body functions adapt slowly, especially when they've been set in a particular pattern for many years. You may adopt a healthier lifestyle in the hope of losing weight and thus reducing your body's production of oestrogen, but find your fat refusing to shift; perhaps you will need to persevere for many months. Don't worry. Natural change is gradual.

Instant answers to health problems are rarely effective in the long term; indeed, they often lead eventually to greater problems. Just as crash diets seem to work wonderfully for a while but leave you more vulnerable to weight problems afterwards, so crash regimes of all sorts can backfire.

Medical treatment is usually designed to produce quick benefits. This is what convinces both doctors and patients that drugs are effective. But when you're dealing with hormone imbalance, this apparently easy answer may not be a good one because the underlying damage due to a faulty lifestyle continues. In health, easy answers are usually illusory: we have to accept personal responsibility for more permanent changes that produce more lasting results.

Hormone imbalance causes both short term distress and long term damage. If your lifestyle affects your hormone cycles so that you suffer from PMT in your twenties, you'll be more susceptible to fibroids and breast disease in your thirties and forties. Then, if you still haven't dealt with the problems effectively, you could confront a difficult menopause. Finally, the same imbalances (attributed to a relative excess of one type of oestrogen) may make you more likely to develop cancers of the breast and ovaries.

Persuading your body to adopt a different hormone balance is inevitably a slow process. You'll probably notice erratic improvements; some months you'll feel better, other months just as bad as before. You might spend a long time on a plateau when you seem to make no progress at all, then, suddenly, everything will function brilliantly. You may get disillusioned or complacent and cease bothering about your hormone health; then a few bad cycles will convince you once again that you can't ignore it.

We all have these ups and downs. Even a health writer like me, who has to look like a shining example of the effectivenss of her own recommendations, will fail to live up to her ideals. I don't worry; if I backslide for a week or a month, I'll pick myself up again. When you've sorted out your life once so that you're making sure your needs are met, you can pick up the threads again more easily later.

It took me about two years to get to the point where I can say that I never suffer from pre-menstrual breast pain or significant period pain. My progress would have been quicker if, when I first decided to sort out my hormones, I'd known what I now know; equally, it would have been better if I had been sufficiently sensible to take all my own good advice! For you, much of the research is done, put together in the book I wish I'd been able to consult; maybe your problems will be more difficult to solve than mine, maybe less severe. But the point is, you can work towards a solution. It's a matter of time and determination.

Our problems are never so bad that we can't do something to make them better; equally, our lives are never so perfect that we can't make improvements. The first step is to make the decision to act, and mean it. From that point on, it's all progress.

Focus on the goal of optimum hormone health. Don't worry about your current state: it'll be different a year from now. Never fear the next phase in your life; you're going to make it a great experience. At this point, you are learning about yourself, about your hormones and about the subtle balance that you have to maintain. You are going to learn how to conduct that marvellous orchestra to create total harmony.

CHAPTER FOUR
The Well-Nourished Woman

Good food is crucial to good health and very few women eat as well as they should. Nutritional deficiency is perhaps the most common reason for hormone problems.

There are many myths about diet, the most pernicious of which is the complacent assurance that anyone who eats a passably varied but conventional diet will be getting all the nutrients they need. This myth is promoted by the many powerful interests in the food production and processing industries and in government, whose main concern seems to be to persuade us to be happy with whatever we're given. Much of the information we receive about food is produced by the public relations organizations of the people who make a lot of money from selling food, and inevitably it's heavily biased in favour of their products.

You are probably conscious of the need for a sensible diet and the chances are that if you already think about your diet, you may doubt that your hormone problems are related to the food you eat. But unless you're very exceptional indeed, you are likely to be suffering from some degree of malnutrition because, quite frankly, it's extremely difficult to avoid it.

If you're overweight, you may imagine you're overnourished. This is just one of the current myths about diet. The reverse is more likely to be true: your weight problem is linked, quite probably, with malnutrition. You, too, need to learn more about good food and how to eat the best food for your body.

Our hormone systems evolved in a world where food was very different from the food we eat today. Our remote ancestresses lived on fresh food that they collected from the environment and these are the foods that we are designed to eat. Nuts, seeds, fruit, roots and insects made up the bulk of the diet, as they still do for the few remaining tribes of hunter-gatherers today. These foods contain a completely different balance of nutrients to those of the typical modern diet.

When women became agriculturalists, the diet changed. Food became more reliable and more plentiful but the balance was often less appropriate to their needs. Changes have continued for thousands of years: now, we have more choices and more access to food than ever before, but few of us consistently make the right choices.

The science of nutrition is a relatively new one. It was only this century that essential trace nutrients and many vitamins were discovered. With continuing study, scientists found that there were a whole series of vitamins; and as research continued, they recognized that many other micro-nutrients were also essential. Now we know that the majority of minerals occurring in nature have a place in maintaining our health and that our diet must contain the full range. The roles of these essential nutrients are still being discovered; even in the last decade, further minerals have been found to be essential to proper hormone balance. No doubt over the next decade yet more links between micro-nutrients and health will be uncovered. Unfortunately, there is a long time-lag between the discovery of a crucial nutrient and acceptance of its importance by the medical profession.

It is now nearly half a century since it was first proposed that hormone imbalance might be linked with malnutrition. In 1931, Dr Biskind, working with American women who suffered from pre-menstrual problems, observed that there were many similarities between his patients' symptoms and those of vitamin B deficiency. He discovered that his patients improved tremendously with vitamin B treatment.

Further research confirmed and extended Dr Biskind's findings. Vitamin E was found to help some menopausal women and vitamin A to improve heavy periods; later, other nutrients including gamma-linolenic acid, magnesium and pyridoxine (vitamin B_6) were all found to reduce problems with PMT. More and more doctors began to use micro-nutrient supplements for hormone imbalances, and many women started to treat themselves with food supplements.

But the underlying problems continued to get worse. Even as vitamin and mineral supplements have grown in popularity, PMT and other signs of hormone imbalance have been rising. The real problem—the nutritional imbalance of our everyday diet—has not been solved.

Unless we eat appropriate, nutrient-rich food every day, we become prone to a whole host of problems. Food that fails to deliver sufficient vitamins, minerals, and other essential nutrients will prove inadequate in many different ways. To pick out one aspect of the insufficiency and correct that on its own is never a satisfactory answer: you never know what other deficiencies you're likely to develop. A much more effective and sensible strategy is to aim for a diet that delivers the whole wide range of nutrients in their natural form, in adequate quantities and in the right proportions for your individual body, so that you don't have to worry about supplements.

But modern food and diets are a minefield. It's easy to get anxious about food and feel that there are so many problems with it, so many things we shouldn't eat and so much contradictory information, that it's impossible to know what to do. Some women, confused by all the warnings, feel so uncertain about food that they imagine they might as well ignore all the experts and just eat whatever is convenient. When everything's taboo, what does it matter?

This chapter shows you ways through the minefield because diet matters very much. Eating well will make you feel healthier in every way and protect you from all types of disease. Eating well maintains all your body functions, keeps your energy levels high and helps you to sleep well at night. And unless you learn to eat well, you will always be vulnerable to hormone problems.

While we all need plenty of good food, our nutrient needs vary with age, lifestyle and individual metabolism. Your own particular health and hormone problems reflect the special needs that you may up until now not have been meeting. The strategy for everyone is to choose a mixed diet, but to concentrate on foods that are especially rich in the nutrients that will help to eliminate the imbalances that you experience and the potential problems that you face. If you have distressing hormone-related symptoms, you will probably benefit from the specific supplements described in this chapter, but when you have achieved a better overall nutritional balance, you may no longer need them.

Whatever your specific requirements, the best diet for hormone health is based on organically grown wholefoods. These are the richest sources of nutrients; organic foods, pro-duced by farmers who do not use artificial chemicals to get artificially high yields, contain higher levels of vitamins and minerals and if you go to the trouble of seeking out organic food, you are less likely to suffer from nutritional deficiencies. Wholefoods are foods in their natural form, containing all the nutritious parts of the plants from which they are derived; processing removes some of the best parts of the food, in many cases substituting chemicals which are often bad for your health. In general, wholefoods, because the outer layers are likely to be intact, are more likely to be brown, while their processed equivalents, because of refining, are white.

The full range of nutrients is necessary to maintain the body's overall metabolic balance and if you are short of any of them, your hormones could suffer indirectly. Some specific nutrients are particularly important. These include the B group vitamins, especially pyridoxine, or B_6; vitamins A, C and E; the essential elements magnesium, potassium, chromium, boron, zinc, iodine and iron, and essential fatty acids. You should ensure that your diet is rich in all these micro-nutrients.

B group vitamins are important in metabolism and in the production of energy from food. They are found in wholegrain products such as bread and brown rice; wheatgerm is a very rich source. Beans and meat, particularly liver, are high in most B group vitamins.

Vitamin B_6 is crucial to normal brain function and stable mood. Deficiency leads to anxiety, depression and insomnia. In recent decades, average consumption of this vitamin has fallen so low that many women are deficient in it; in addition, for reasons that are described in the next chapter, our requirements have risen. Taking oral contraceptives, drinking alcohol, and smoking all increase your need for this vitamin. Good sources include oily fish, egg yolk, whole grains, nuts (especially walnuts), seeds, bananas and avocados.

If you are contemplating pregnancy or if you are already pregnant, another B group vitamin, folic acid, is very important for your baby's health. Folic acid deficiency in early pregnancy can lead to nervous system malformations such as spina bifida. Make sure you get sufficient folic acid by eating plenty of green leafy vegetables, avocados, almonds, walnuts and oranges.

Vitamin A can be helpful for women with heavy periods and it's an important anti-cancer vitamin. If you eat enough fresh vegetables and fruit, your intake should be adequate; taking supplements of vitamin A can cause dangerous side-effects. Good sources include carrots, green leafy vegetables, egg yolk, fruit with orange-coloured flesh such as apricots and peaches, and oily fish.

Vitamin C is necessary for the production of sex hormones. It is found in very high concentration in the adrenal glands, which produce progesterone, testosterone, and oestrogens. During and after menopause, when the adrenal glands take over an increasing role in sex hormone production, it is essential to keep your vitamin C intake up. Vitamin C can also help women with heavy periods. It is used up especially fast when you are exposed to pollution, when you smoke, and when you are fighting infection, so make sure you increase your consumption of foods rich in this vitamin if any of these conditions apply to you.

Vitamin C is found in most fresh vegetables, especially watercress, broccoli and new potatoes; in citrus and berry fruits such as oranges, grapefruit, strawberries and raspberries; in pineapple and melon and in most tropical fruits. Both storage and cooking reduce the amount of vitamin C in food so make sure it is as fresh as possible.

Vitamin E has been called the 'sex' hormone, for without it, male animals, from rats to men, became impotent. It is essential for fertility; it is also known as tocopherol, which is derived from the Greek word for 'childbearing'. It is important throughout life, but it seems to be especially beneficial for reducing menopausal symptoms. If you have long-standing digestive problems, you could be deficient in vitamin E.

Sunflower seeds and sunflower oil are very good sources of vitamin E. Other nuts, particularly almonds, hazelnuts and peanuts, are good too and should form a regular part of your diet. Avocados, sweet potatoes and wild blackberries are other valuable sources.

Magnesium is probably the most important of the minerals for good hormone balance and it's the one in which you are most likely to be deficient. Everyone should aim to eat magnesium-rich foods every day; if you suffer from PMT, sore breasts or period pain, you may need magnesium supplements. If you are short of magnesium, your body will be unable to use vitamin B_6 and you will show signs of B_6 deficiency such as poor skin condition. Many women who try B_6 on its own to relieve PMT find that it has little effect because they also need magnesium to get the benefit. Magnesium is crucial in maintaining the hormone balance that will keep you healthy during pregnancy, and in keeping your bones strong well into old age.

Magnesium deficiency is almost universal because modern farming methods produce food that's very low in magnesium. Ironically, many farmers are well aware of this; farm animals are given magnesium supplements because agricultural experts acknowledge that pasture and feedstuffs grown with chemical fertilizers do not contain sufficient magnesium to maintain animal health. The effects of deficiency show up most severely during pregnancy, when animals develop toxaemia and can die or lose their young.

Human food is deficient in magnesium for the same reason; yet oddly enough, the Ministry of Agriculture, Fisheries and Food denies that food produced for our consumption is deficient in minerals. Why they think that humans need less of this mineral than farm animals, I cannot understand. However, farmers who feed their animals organic food, produced without nitrate fertilizers, find that supplements are unnecessary; and the same is often true of people.

Magnesium is essential to metabolism. Its chief function is to 'activate' enzymes, especially those related to energy production; if you tend to feel tired all the time, you will find that increasing your magnesium intake will be particularly helpful. Magnesium deficiency during pregnancy can cause toxaemia. Women with PMT are also usually short of magnesium, and the high magnesium demands of pregnancy may explain why PMT can start after childbirth.

The best sources of magnesium are nuts, especially almonds, brazils, cashews and hazelnuts. Organic whole grain products, wheatgerm, tofu (bean curd) and seaweed are also rich in this mineral.

Potassium is linked with hormone effects in two ways: it is crucial for water balance and for nerve function. If you suffer from water-retention, more potassium in your diet will help.

Potassium works with sodium in the body and the correct balance of these two chemically similar elements is important to health. Unfortunately, our diet does not provide the right balance because we add sodium (contained in ordinary salt, baking powder and other food additives) while potassium is lost through cooking and processing. The relative excess of sodium makes the shortage of potassium more severe.

To increase your potassium intake, eat more raw fruit and vegetables—they all contain potassium. Seaweeds, sunflower seeds, wheatgerm, nuts and raisins, bananas, avocados, green vegetables and potatoes are particularly high in this element. If you decrease your sodium intake by avoiding salty or processed foods at the same time as increasing your potassium intake, you will double the benefit.

Chromium, in contrast to potassium, is present in the body in tiny quantities, but it is nevertheless essential. Chromium is necessary for blood sugar control. Many pregnant women and women with PMT have borderline diabetic symptoms which can be eliminated with chromium. If you suffer from sugar or carbohydrate cravings, increasing your chromium intake could be the answer. Ironically, if you give into your cravings and eat sweets, your chromium excretion will increase, making the problem worse!

By far the best natural source of chromium is yeast. Liver, wholemeal bread, wheatgerm and beef are also good sources.

Iron is essential for the blood. Deficiency causes anaemia, one sign of which is that blood-rich membranes like the insides of our eyelids turn pale. As you'd expect, iron is particularly important for women who have heavy periods; indeed iron deficiency itself can cause heavy periods and the problem gets worse with each monthly loss of blood. It is very important for pregnant women, who need both to produce large amounts of iron-rich tissue to sustain the pregnancy, and to supply the baby with iron.

Although iron does not seem to be directly involved in hormone production and metabolism, monthly blood loss means that women regularly lose some iron from their bodies. Iron deficiency is a common cause of lack of physical energy and recurrent infections such as thrush.

The foods richest in iron are kelp, yeast, molasses, pumpkin and sunflower seeds, wheat germ and liver; nuts and raisins are also good sources. The green colour of leafy vegetables and the red colour of meat are both due to iron, but the body cannot always absorb this iron; eating spinach, for example, won't improve your iron status because the oxalic acid it also contains prevents absorption. The iron in meat is more readily available, but vegetarians should not be unduly concerned about risking deficiency by refusing meat; they are actually less prone to anaemia than meat-eaters.

One problem with iron is that absorption is very sensitive to the way we mix our food and drink. If you have vitamin C with your iron—a grapefruit to start your meal, or new potatoes with your meat, for example—you will absorb more. If you have tea or a soft drink with, or within an hour of, your meal, you will absorb considerably less. Some people will be able to cure iron deficiency problems simply by substituting a glass of natural fruit juice for the tea or soft drink they formerly had with meals.

Iron deficiency may also be due to internal bleeding and if this is the case, taking more will not solve the problem. Ulcers are often to blame; frequent taking of aspirin and similar drugs is probably the most important cause.

A simple and useful way to get your iron status checked is to become a blood donor. If your blood is low in iron, you will not be allowed to make a donation—and you'll know you need to take action to increase your intake or absorption. If the nurse allows you to go ahead and donate, you can be sure you can spare the iron!

Zinc is involved in a wide range of metabolic processes in the body. It is crucial for normal growth, cell division and tissue repair, for the development of sex organs in men, and for the establishment of a regular menstrual cycle in adolescent girls. During pregnancy, the growing baby makes enormous demands on the mother's zinc reserves; some experts believe that the zinc deficiency this causes can contribute to morning sickness. Zinc is necessary for healthy skin and bones; zinc-deficient women are more likely to develop stretch marks on their skin and to suffer osteoporosis after menopause.

The best source of zinc, by far, is oysters. Other zinc-rich foods include red meat, nuts, and organic whole grains.

Boron is essential for normal levels of oestrogen in post-menopausal women; a high boron diet can double the oestrogen content of the blood and thus protect you from osteoporosis, vaginal dryness and other oestrogen deficiency symptoms. Boron has only recently been identified as a nutrient, and its role is not yet fully known; however, it's likely that a mineral that is so beneficial to the hormone systems of older women is also necessary for younger women. Plant foods, especially fresh vegetables and fruit, are high in boron. If you eat both fruit and vegetables every day, your body's boron needs are likely to be adequately met.

Iodine is another trace element known to be implicated in hormone-related conditions. Iodine is crucial to the activity of the thyroid gland and when thyroid hormones are in short supply, women develop PMT. Breast cancer is more common among women with thyroid problems. The links between thyroid hormones, PMT and breast cancer seem to involve oestrogen, but the details of the picture have yet to emerge. What is clear, however, is that a high iodine intake can improve hormone balance.

Iodine is found in fish and seafood: haddock, halibut, sardines and shellfish all contain large quantities. Other, less rich, sources include liver, pineapple, eggs, peanuts and wholewheat products.

Essential fatty acids (EFAs) are the final group of nutrients that are essential for hormone health. Both pre-menstrual problems and period pain can improve dramatically with an increased intake of EFAs. They have many roles to play in the body, but one that is particularly relevant to women, is their contribution to the production and metabolism of prostaglandins, which are involved in period pain and general discomfort.

The best-known source of EFA is evening primrose, but it is not usually necessary to increase your intake of this nutrient by supplementing your diet with evening primrose oil. EFAs are also found in wheatgerm (especially wheatgerm oil), seeds, particularly linseed (sold as Linusit Gold in health shops), and cold-water fish such as herring, salmon and pilchards.

EFA deficiency is common because of the effects of food processing, but also because other dietary fats (especially the fat in margarine and commercial baked goods like biscuits) increase our need for EFAs. The next chapter explains more about this problem.

Looking back through this list of essential nutrients and their sources, you will see that certain foods crop up again and again.

These are shown in Table 1, below.

Table 1

Super-nutrient foods

1. Nuts and seeds
2. Whole grains and wheatgerm
3. Liver*
4. Avocado
5. Green vegetables (peas, beans and leafy greens)
6. Potatoes and carrots
7. Fruit
8. Food from the sea—fish and seaweed

* Note: The liver you eat must come from organically farmed animals. The liver concentrates both nutrients and poisons; so if animals have been exposed to hormones, drugs and chemicals as all conventionally produced animals are, the liver could contain dangerously high levels of these substances.

Top of the above list are nuts and seeds. Most people regard these as snack foods, but this underestimates their importance; you should treat them as essential parts of your diet, eating 2 to 4 ounces (50–100g) of a variety of nuts and seeds every day. Nuts and seeds provide high-quality protein as well as many micro-nutrients and you can use them to replace meat in your diet.

Try to avoid salted, roasted nuts: they're much better raw. Nuts are extremely versatile; eat them with meals, in nut roasts, muesli, salads, curries or vegetarian dishes; in sauces (try walnut sauce with your vegetables, experiment with peanut sauce in Indonesian recipes), and in sweets. Use nut butters on your bread—almond, hazelnut and cashew butters are delicious, but ordinary peanut butter is good too—and chew a handful of seeds when you want a quick snack.

We should not be surprised at the value of nuts. Our ancestral grandmothers would have relied heavily on them to keep their families going. Nuts and seeds are the only natural foods that keep for long periods, and the landscape of thousands of years ago contained many more trees. We are foolish if we forget our ancestral diet and ignore one of its major components.

Next on the list are wholegrain products. Grains form the staple food of most countries but their nutritional value has been much reduced by chemical farming, refining and processing. Wheatgerm, which is removed from grain to produce white flour products, contains the highest nutrient concentration; it is a valuable food supplement and you can sprinkle it on cereals, soups, crumbles or yoghurt. Enrich your baking by adding wheatgerm to organic wholewheat flour. Always buy organic bread and pasta if you can, or bake your own using organic wholemeal flour (I recommend Dove's Farm), because pesticides adhere to the bran and the germ in wholewheat flour and you can get a frighteningly high dose with bread derived from conventionally-grown wheat.

A minority of women with severe hormone problems are allergic to wheat. If you have changed your diet and way of life in accordance with the recommendations in the book and you continue to have problems. Chapter eight gives further information. You'll find you have to replace the nutritional value of wheat with other grains, particularly organic brown rice and buckwheat.

Liver is the next of our super-nutrient foods. The liver acts as a storage organ for the body, concentrating a host of nutrients. It's a highly metabolically active organ, chock-full of enzymes and co-enzymes which are rich in micro-nutrients.

Regrettably, this super-food is not what it used to be. The liver also concentrates drugs, hormone implant residues, poisons and pesticides because it's the body's major de-toxifying organ. So if you eat liver from conventionally farmed animals, the poisons in it could outbalance the benefit you enjoy from its stored nutrients. You can solve this problem by buying organic liver: it's more expensive but it tastes better and it's better for you. If your local butcher doesn't stock it, find an organic butcher in your local area or get it from Wholefood (24 & 31 Paddington Street, London W1).

Vegetables are the next major item on the top-foods list. First comes the avocado, in a class of its own. Have you been avoiding avocado because of its high-calorie image or because it's expensive? Think again! Its nutrient value is exceptional and that makes it both good for you and good value for money. Eat avocado in your salads, mashed in dips, or on its own with home-made vinaigrette or shrimps.

Green vegetables are also marvellous, but of course you knew that! Most of us have been told to eat our greens since we were small and too few people eat enough. British families eat fewer vegetables than any other Europeans and one result is an exceptionally high rate of birth malformations and subnormal children. Your dinner plate should be piled high with fresh vegetables, as much as you can tolerate, and in as much variety as possible.

Potatoes play an important part in our diet. Eat as many as you like, as often as you like. Boil or bake them, don't fry them; if you eat chips, you're doing yourself a disservice. Heated fats—especially re-heated fats—are associated with long term hormone-related cancers. If your potatoes are not organically grown do not eat the peel. The next chapter explains the hazards of chemical-treated and fried potatoes. Buy new potatoes whenever they are available and go for flavour; this is your best guide to quality.

Seaweed is used as a vegetable by some of the healthiest populations in the world, particularly the Japanese. Experiment with seaweed in your diet; many types are available from wholefood shops and Chinese supermarkets.

Fruit should have a special place in every woman's diet: delicious fruit is also health-giving. Bananas, oranges, soft fruit and tropical fruits such as mangoes are especially nutritious. Apples and pears should be peeled unless you know they are unsprayed. Aim to eat about a pound of raw fruit every day.

Fish is better for hormone health than meat. Oily fish like herring and pilchards are especially valuable because many nutrients are found in association with the fat in their flesh. Unfortunately, the pollution of our seas means that the health value of some once-excellent fish is not what it was; the feeding grounds of eels, for example, are usually heavily contaminated with industrial waste. Deep-water fish like cod is the safest. Wild salmon and sea trout is good, but make sure it is wild before you buy. Fish farming is becoming as suspect as other types of farming, with excessively large populations living in confined spaces where disease spreads so that farmers use drugs and chemicals to protect the economic value of their crop.

Food Supplements

There is mounting evidence that women with hormone imbalance problems can benefit from supplementing their diets with specific nutrients. Doctors in different clinics tend to concentrate on the nutrients they believe in, and despite the rather simplistic approach of using one or two supplements at a time, some good results have been achieved. By putting together the supplements that may help or that work well together, you can increase the benefits.

Gamma-linolenic acid, an uncommon essential fatty acid, was accidently discovered to be valuable for women with menstrual problems by Dr David Horrobin when he was working on other health problems in a Montreal clinic. Women reported that their PMT improved when they took GLA in the form of evening primrose oil. Dr Horrobin's work was extended by Dr Michael Brush, who had been studying vitamin B_6 at St Thomas's Hospital in London. Dr Brush had already found that vitamin B_6 therapy (50–200 mg daily during the second half of the menstrual cycle) reduced the distress of PMT for about 70 per cent of his patients; GLA was helpful for many of the remaining 30 per cent.

Other doctors, dealing with a variety of hormone problems, discovered that other vitamins and minerals could also be very useful. The most influential individual in the field is probably Dr Guy Abraham, who studied PMT in patients at a Californian gynaecological clinic. He helped clarify the roles of vitamins C and E, magnesium and zinc.

Dr Abraham's work was extended and developed by Dr Alan Stewart at the Women's Nutritional Advisory Centre in Hove, Sussex. There, a wide range of food supplements are used to help women with a variety of health problems, and, with the co-operation of manufacturers Nature's Best, some very effective formulations have been developed to enable women to treat themselves.

While the ideal solution is to get all the nourishment we need from food, we can't always manage this. Extra doses of particular nutrients may be necessary to get your body's balance right. There are many possible reasons for this. You may have been running short of essential nutrients for years, or been through a period of increased nutrient requirements. You may have a problem with absorption or excretion of particular nutrients or an individual biochemical makeup that means your requirements are unusually high. You may have been exposed to chemicals that reduce your body's ability to use nutrients or you may be unable to break lifetime habits that increase nutrient demands. Under such circumstances, your hormone problems may not resolve themselves without the use of specific food supplements.

However, using specific supplements is not as straightforward as it may seem. Picking a product that will work requires understanding, both of your own problem and of the nature of dietary supplements. There are many reports in the medical literature of people damaging themselves with unwise supplementation, especially when they use mega-doses of vitamins or minerals. Most nutrients, taken in excess, can be dangerous; more is not necessarily better for you. The vogue for mega-supplementation is not based on any physiological wisdom.

Never take mega-doses of vitamins or minerals. High doses can be toxic. If you take too much of any mineral, you will upset your body's overall balance and you could create other deficiencies. For example, excess zinc produces copper deficiency, and vice-versa. Too much vitamin B_6 (over 200 mg daily for most people) can cause neurological symptoms. Too much vitamin C may lead to kidney problems. So stick to the doses recommended on the labels of the containers: more is definitely not better. Best of all, keep your supplement needs to the absolute minimum by eating a varied, nutrient-dense diet. Food is naturally balanced; it's the best nutrient source you can get.

Supplementation is a controversial area. Some doctors will deny all the evidence and maintain that you don't need any supplements. Others accept that they can work, but fail to realize that the form of supplement you use can be important. My experience, reading and observation has convinced me that the form such supplementation takes can be crucial.

If you need extra iron because you have excessive bleeding or you are pregnant, you wouldn't try to chew iron filings or lick the rust from an old pan. You don't expect iron in these forms to do you any good. That intuition is right: nutrients in food are not the same as the simple chemicals they contain. Natural minerals in food are bound up in complex organic molecules akin to the molecules in our bodies; iron in green plants, for example, is mainly found in the chlorophyll, a substance rather similar to haemoglobin. Our bodies evolved in parallel with it so our systems are designed to use it.

A good way to overcome any problem with supplements is by using naturally-occurring substances that are especially high in the nutrients you need. It is virtually impossible to overdose on these special foods. Natural food supplements include wheatgerm, kelp, linseed and evening primrose oil.

Wheatgerm is rich in B group vitamins and vitamin E. Add wheatgerm to your diet if you're pregnant, or if you suffer from breast problems, PMT or menopausal flushes. Sprinkle it on cereals, eat it with yoghurt, and add it to any flour you use in baking. Wheatgerm oil is nutritious and delicious; add it to salad dressings for an extra-special nutty flavour.

Kelp tablets are concentrated forms of seaweed (see above). They are very rich in a wide range of minerals and include a high proportion of iodine. Kelp tablets can be particularly beneficial if you have breast problems. Use them to keep your nutritional level high during pregnancy.

Evening primrose oil is one of the richest known sources of essential fatty acids in a readily-usable form. Try supplements for period problems of all kinds, especially if you also suffer from dry skin or allergies.

Fish liver oils also contain high levels of vitamins, minerals and essential fatty acids; they have been used for many years as food supplements. Although I am sure that these were excellent a few decades ago, I do not recommend these oils now because I am unhappy about the concentration of toxic substances in fish livers. Both toxic metals such as mercury and synthetic poisons such as PCBs are concentrated in fish livers; I was shocked when I saw the Ministry of Agriculture Fishery Research Centre figures for pollutants in raw cod liver.

If you decide to use supplements, it makes sense to use a form close to those occuring naturally in food. When supplements are ineffective or produce unpleasant side-effects, it's often because they are not in forms that the body can easily use. For example, ferrous sulphate, an inorganic chemical compound containing iron, is often prescribed for anaemia, but it is poorly absorbed and can cause digestive problems. In ferrous gluconate, iron is chemically bound to an organic molecule (gluconic acid, a

Table 2

Nutrients for hormone health

Minerals/Trace elements	Boron	Calcium	Chromium	Iodine
Problem/Status				
PMT			*	
Heavy periods				
Painful periods		*		
No periods				
Pregnant	*	**	**	*
Menopausal[1]	*	*	*	*
Post-menopause[2]	*	*	*	

Vitamins/EFAs	A	B group	B$_6$	C
Problem/Status				
PMT		*	**	*
Heavy periods	*		*	*
Painful periods			*	
No periods	*	*	*	*
Pregnant	*	*	*	*
Menopausal[1]		*	*	
Post-menopausal[2]		*		*

[1] Experiencing symptoms such as hot flushes

[2] One year or more after periods have ceased

Iron	Magnesium	Potassium	Selenium	Zinc
	**	*		
**				*
	*			*
	*			*
*	**	*	*	*
	*	*	*	
	*		*	

E	EFAS	Bioflavonoids
*	*	
		*
*	*	
*	*	
*	*	*
*	*	
	*	

relative of glucose), which makes it less troublesome to the digestive system.

When you're selecting mineral supplements, go for organic forms every time. Read the label, looking out for key words like 'chelate' (pronounced keelate). This is the technical term for an inorganic chemical (such as iron) bound in a substance that you're likely to be able to absorb.

The crucial question is, which supplements will help you? One way of side-stepping it is to use a multi-vitamin and mineral supplement which should meet all your needs, whatever they are. Again, choose carefully! Make sure that it contains all the minerals in Table 2 overleaf, checking that they are in organic forms, and all the vitamins. One excellent multi-vitamin and mineral supplement is *Health Insurance Plus*, from Nature's Best, Freepost P.O. Box 1, Tunbridge Wells TN2 3EQ (0892 34143). Table 2 lists the nutrients in which you're most likely to be deficient.

Using separate supplements to boost your intake of specific nutrients requires more thought than just taking a general-purpose multi-nutrient tablet. Many nutrients work in conjunction with others: for example, zinc and iron are best absorbed with vitamin C, while magnesium requires adequate B_6. It may be that you are getting enough vitamin C from a diet high in fruit and fresh vegetables and you don't need a supplement to enhance your mineral absorption, but this is something you should consider carefully.

Some supplements are designed for hormone problems and contain a limited, yet specific range of nutrients designed to help with particular problems. Nature's Best has worked closely with Dr Guy Abraham, a specialist in the treatment of PMT, to produce *Optivite for Women*. It contains nutrients known to help with menstrual problems. Another Nature's Best product is *Sugar Factor*, for people with sugar and carbohydrate cravings. Again, this can be very helpful in controlling PMT.

Other manufacturers, such as Quest, Seven Seas and Health-crafts also produce chelated nutrient supplements, although to my knowledge none has developed supplements as specifically valuable to women with hormone imbalance symptoms as some of those described above. However, you may not be able to get Nature's Best products from your local chemist or health food shop.

While supplements can make an obvious difference to the way

you feel in the first month you use them, it may be three months before their full effects are apparent. Don't give up this approach if you don't feel any immediate benefit; allow your body time to establish a better nutritional balance.

You may find that you don't have to continue with supplements once you are on an even keel and you've adjusted your lifestyle to maintain a better balance. Plentiful good food and adequate exercise could be all you need once you've made up the nutrient shortfall that has developed over years. So try cutting down the supplements gradually when you feel your diet is sufficiently balanced. You can always re-introduce them when you're under stress or symptoms begin to return.

I find that a minimal level of supplementation (50 mg chelated magnesium on most days) is usually sufficient for my needs. If I'm under pressure, I'll add 50 mg B_6 daily for the second half of the month. When I get carbohydrate cravings, I'll substitute Sugar Factor, which contains both of these nutrients along with chromium and other vitamins, for my separate supplements. I go by the way I feel.

After a period of experimentation, you'll come to know the effects of particular supplements on your metabolism. You may find that symptoms return if you cut back too far—for example, I find I get breast problems and period pain when my magnesium levels fall. For you, other nutrients may be more important: for example, your body may be particularly poor at metabolising essential fatty acids, so that you get pain unless you take evening primrose oil. Experience is the best guide. Never assume that because a supplement worked wonders for your friend, it is bound to be the best thing for you; but equally, don't dismiss it because it wasn't the answer for her. Remember that we are all different.

Our needs change over the years, as Table 2 indicates. A different set of nutrients become important with the hormone hiatus of menopause; you may find that vitamin E, which had no apparent effect when you were younger, is just what you need to control hot flushes. If your periods get heavier, you should look to your iron status, whereas if they get lighter, you may be able to give up the extra iron you'd been taking.

You may wish to use hair analysis to find out more about your nutrient status. This can provide valuable insights when it is done by a reputable firm but it is not always reliable. Excellent results can be obtained, through a doctor's referral, to Biolab, of

The Stone House, 9 Weymouth Street, London W1N 3FF but this company does not deal directly with the public.

If you try hair analysis, the following tips will improve the technique's accuracy. Cut a lock of hair from the back of the head, as close to the scalp as possible; an inch or two will be sufficient. Perms, colourings, conditioners and some shampoos—especially anti-dandruff shampoo—can distort the result. A competent laboratory will ask about the products you use on your hair and take these into account.

You may well wonder why you should need supplements if you take care to choose a varied diet. The reason is that today's environment and modern food production make a sufficiently nutritious diet hard to achieve. Unless you eat plenty of organic food, you are likely to be undernourished; and even those who are able to live on organic food may run into problems for reasons described in the next chapter.

For those who do not make the effort to eat organic food, malnutrition is now, in my opinion, inevitable. Hormone problems are symptoms of borderline malnutrition and modern farming methods are largely responsible for this. These methods have been promoted by successive governments all of which have had cheap food policies. This has led to the impoverishment of our food through subsidies on growing methods that do not produce the most nourishing food.

The best food is rarely the cheapest. You may have to spend a higher proportion of your income on food. Cheap food is an illusion: you pay with your health and we all pay through damage to the environment. We have to accept that good food costs more in both terms of money and time than we may have been led to believe. Over recent years, we have been sold increasingly shoddy goods; now, more and more people are rejecting junk and looking for food that tastes as good as it did 30 years ago.

Modern farming relies on a small group of chemicals to produce heavy yields from the fields. The same chemicals are used on the land, whether for arable farming and vegetable or grain production, or grassland farming and meat production; these are nitrogen, potassium and phosphorus. When these elements are plentiful, crops grow quickly and grass looks wonderfully green. The problem is that these fast-growing crops are deficient in the other minerals that they would naturally contain and which we need for our well-balanced diet.

Some of the micro-nutrient deficiencies in our food occur because the necessary minerals have been exhausted from the soil by successive crops. Others develop because high levels of the minerals used in commercial fertilizers interfere with the uptake of other minerals by plants. For example, when farmers use a lot of nitrates on their fields, the plants are not able to take up adequate magnesium—even if it is present in the soil. So the food that is produced is deficient in magnesium before it even leaves the farm. Processing and cooking will then remove a proportion of what remains. Predictably, magnesium deficiency is very common indeed, and it is one cause of hormone problems.

Processing and storage further depletes our food of nutritional value. Levels of some vitamins, for example vitamin C, decline rapidly in store. Unfortunately, our distribution and marketing systems are designed to allow food to be kept for increasingly long periods before we buy it. It may look fresh, but the chances are it isn't.

Happily, good food is re-appearing in the shops. It is labelled 'organic' and it's usually marked with the Soil Association Symbol of Organic Quality. It is uncontaminated with sprays, produced without damage to the environment, and it is the richest in both flavour and nutrients. Once you make a policy of buying organic, you'll never go back to chemical rubbish if you can possibly avoid it. It just doesn't taste good enough.

Buying organic has other implications too. It is part of the fight against the chemical pollution of our environment. Organic farming does not lead to the pollution of drinking water with nitrates and pesticides; it is a way of farming that cherishes the environment and the creatures which share the land with us. It allows wild animals to flourish because it does not poison natural food chains with chemical toxins. And it allows wild flowers to bloom in beautiful profusion because it does not involve the use of herbicides which kill every plant except the farmer's crop. So if you care about the natural world, you can help preserve it by buying organic food.

If you care about animals, you should only buy organic meat and eggs. Organic farmers do not keep their animals in over-crowded sheds; all animals are free-range and they do not receive any drugs or antibiotics unless these are essential to treat illness. With this gentle way of farming, illness is rare; animals stay healthy when they are treated as they should be. The meat from these unstressed animals is tastier and better for you.

By eating organic, you will be getting nutrient-rich foods. Organic produce has higher levels of micro-nutrients so you are much less likely to run into deficiency problems. This is something that the Ministry of Agriculture ignores when it supports chemical farming. Oddly enough, ministry experts and vets acknowledge that animals fed on pasture produced by conventional means with fertilizers and herbicides become mineral deficient and must be given supplements. Yet they pretend that humans do not suffer the same way when their food is similarly impoverished! Find out more by joining the Soil Association, 86 Colston Street, Bristol BS1 5BB (0272 290661) or by writing off for some of their information leaflets.

Food processing compounds the problem. It removes nutrients, substituting junk. Any highly processed food—like white flour products and sugar—is deficient in nutrients. The less you do to your food, the better. When you can eat food raw, do so; a salad a day is very good for your health. Many people believe that living food—raw vegetables in particular—is particularly nourishing. My experience certainly bears this out but there is not yet any scientific proof of its special value. All I can say is that sprouted grains and beans, eaten raw in salads, do wonders for the way I feel.

Sprouting is the easiest way to obtain fresh, cheap, nutritious food. Almost any dried beans can be sprouted, but mung beans are the easiest and most popular. Sprout them in a large jar in your airing cupboard or any other warm place. My method is to put a handful of beans in a large coffee jar and soak them in water for 24 hours. Then rinse them in fresh water, pour off the water, and leave them to sprout with a loose top on the jar. On each of the next few days, rinse them once or twice until they've grown sprouts about an inch long: they are then ready to eat. Don't leave them to grow too long: once they have a pair of green leaves, their flavour deteriorates.

You may feel that it's not worth while taking the trouble to sprout your own beans, going out of your way to find shops that sell organic food, and doing all the preparation work that's involved in eating natural foods. You may say that your diet is varied and balanced already, and that people in Britain, according to government spokespersons, do not tend to suffer from significant nutrient deficiencies. But if you have problems with your hormones—indeed, if you are in less than tip-top health in any way—you should pay attention to the nutrient value of your food.

If you've ever done any gardening, or even looked after houseplants, you'll know the difference that feeding plants properly makes. Without muck, or compost, or seaweed fertilizer, your plants will probably hang on and grow slowly. But if you feed them well, they will look luxurious, green and healthy, and resist disease. It's the same with people. Humans are immensely adaptable and capable of surviving all sorts of hardship and a very poor level of nourishment, but these conditions do not allow us to thrive. The difference between thriving and managing somehow is the difference that good food can make. And keeping the subtle balance of your hormones at an optimum level demands that all the nutrients your body needs are also at an optimum level.

Busy mothers may complain that they don't have the time or energy to go to a lot of trouble with food. In my opinion, they should re-think their priorities. Food is crucial to health—not just your own health, but the health of future generations. By bringing up your daughters on the most nourishing food you can get, you will reduce the risk of illness when they grow up.

Your children may react against you, selecting junk as a form of rebellion, especially during adolescence. I have noticed that these children will revert to choosing good food after a few years when they notice how much worse they feel when they fail to feed themselves well. Children imitate their parents and learn their eating habits from them. Make sure you protect your daughters by teaching them the best way of eating at an early age.

CHAPTER FIVE
Pollution and the Anti-Nutrient Problem

Eating the right food is part of the solution to the nutrition problem; avoiding substances that harm us is equally important. Exposure to pollution and chemicals increases our susceptibility to hormone imbalance problems. Our bodies were not designed to cope with the chemical input of the modern world.

When we evolved, our ancestresses drank only water but today's women choose tea, coffee, soft drinks, cocktails. Our ancestressses had access to little salt so they seasoned food with woodash, herbs, and occasionally honey; we use salt, sugar, flavour enhancers and chemical additives. We are exposed to hazardous substances, from pesticides to preservatives, that did not exist until recently. Our ancestors, like third-world women today, suffered from malnutrition due to simple lack of food; we suffer malnutrition amid plenty because of the contamination and impoverishment of our food. From Birmingham to Beijing, women are exposed to substances that the people from whom we descended never encountered. Some of these substances act as anti-nutrients.

Anti-nutrients interfere with the absorption, metabolism or transport of nutrients in the body. The more we are exposed to anti-nutrients, the more nutrients we need to counterbalance their effects. If we have too much of some of these substances in our bodies, it may be impossible to achieve a healthy hormone balance.

The concept of the anti-nutrient is relatively new; until recently, it was assumed that if a food contained a nutrient, our bodies would be able to use it effectively. This is the basis on which the government's Recommended Daily Allowances (RDAs) are worked out. But when you are exposed to anti-nutrients, you may need far larger quantities of some nutrients than you normally would.

The average diet in Britain and most developed countries is heavily loaded with anti-nutrients. Some are the products of conventional farming, which relies on chemicals to control pests and produce perfect-looking, standard produce which can be easily harvested. After harvest, the spraying continues, with more chemicals needed to keep crops looking good and prevent decay. Virtually all our food is sprayed many times before it reaches the shop. British potatoes and onions, for example, get such a liberal dose of growth inhibitor to prevent them from sprouting that our onions have for years been rejected by the French because of the chemical residues they contain.

Pesticides, biocides of all kinds, and chemicals which affect ripening, sprayed on growing crops and on to food in store, are poisons which have to be made harmless in our bodies. Sometimes we are unable to excrete them and these poisonous chemicals and their breakdown products accumulate in our bodies, disrupting enzyme function and throwing our bio-chemistry out of balance. Poisonous chemicals pollute the air we breathe, our water, and, to a greater or lesser degree, all the food we eat. They are ubiquitous. We cannot avoid them completely but we can significantly reduce the quantity we take in.

Drugs, too, can have anti-nutrient effects. In addition, the longer you take a drug, the more likely it is to cause problems for you. This is true of many medicines, including contraceptive drugs, but it also applies to our most common social drugs—alcohol, coffee and tea. Tobacco smoke is another everyday pollutant that increases our nutrient requirements. Fortunately, we are usually able to choose whether to expose ourselves to these substances.

As with many aspects of health, we vary tremendously in our susceptibility to chemical hazards. Your body may be able to cope with substances that throw your friend's totally out of kilter; but you could find, as I have done, that some seemingly intractable symptoms will respond quickly when you pay attention to anti-nutrient intake.

The most pervasive anti-nutrients for most of us are in our everyday food and drink. Some of the substances that we take in most regularly can interfere with nutrient absorption in the digestive system.

Tea is one example. In England, women and tea-drinking are almost inseparable and many women drink tea both with and between meals. Unfortunately, chemicals in tea reduce the absorption of iron and zinc from food. This is especially important if you are a heavy tea-drinker at meal-times. Tea-drinking causes or exacerbates many hormone-related problems; probably the causes are more complex than simple interference with nutrient absorption. However, research has shown that women who drink more than four cups of tea each day suffer more PMT symptoms than those who drink less. This effect has been demonstrated both in China and in England.

Substituting coffee for tea will not help matters. Coffee has been convincingly linked with breast problems, especially fibrocystic breast disease (painful, lumpy breasts) and pre-menstrual breast tenderness. It can aggravate anxiety, palpitations and nervous tension, all of which will be more severe both pre-menstrually and during the menopause if you drink a lot of coffee. In addition, coffee, like tea, reduces absorption of zinc and iron when you drink it with meals.

Coffee and tea contain stimulant drugs (caffeine and theobromine) but substituting decaffeinated tea and coffee isn't likely to help much. Caffeine is only part of the problem; these drinks contain a whole cocktail of chemicals which affect many parts of our bodies. To make matters worse, they act as diuretics, causing our kidneys to filter more water from the blood. While this will make us urinate more often, it doesn't help reduce water retention or bloating because it makes you want to drink more. With the extra loss of urine, you will lose minerals such as magnesium and potassium. The diuretic effect became obvious to me when I realized that a cup of ordinary tea in the evening makes me get up in the night, whereas a herb tea such as rosehip or camomile does not disturb my sleep in this way.

Giving up tea and coffee can be difficult. Many people are addicted to them and going cold turkey can cause headaches and depression. Fortunately these symptoms pass in a couple of days. What is more difficult to cope with is the social nature of tea and coffee drinking: even if you know it's bad for you, it can be very hard to resist saying yes to a cuppa when the pot's on the table and everyone else is having some.

The best solution is to try a variety of drinks such as herbal teas and discover the types you really like. Keep them handy so that when somebody suggests tea, you can immediately say, 'No thanks, but I'd love lemon verbena' (or apple juice, or whatever you fancy at the time). This isn't a lot of trouble for anyone—

though I find that some people really do try to undermine my resolve! Addicts are notorious for putting pressure on those who say no to their chosen drug.

Giving up tea and coffee drinking makes a real difference to the way I feel. I'm more alert and less likely to suffer pre-menstrual symptoms. I found it relatively easy to give up coffee; someday I'll manage to refuse tea every time—I wish I didn't like it quite so much!

Alcohol acts as an anti-nutrient by increasing our need for B-group vitamins including B_1, vitamin D, and the minerals magnesium, zinc and calcium. Even social drinking has this effect, while heavy drinking can cause serious malnutrition. In addition, alcohol damages the liver, leading directly to problems with hormone metabolism. Women are more vulnerable than men to alcohol damage and any woman who has hormone imbalance symptoms should drink very little alcohol.

Tea, coffee and alcohol are not the only substances that can alter mineral absorption and excretion. Chemical additives in food and drink can have similar effects.

Phosphates and polyphosphates (E450, 544 and 545), common constituents of a wide range of products including soft drinks, cheeses, processed meats, frozen fish products, and even whole frozen chickens and hams, are believed to interfere with nutrient absorption by interfering with the action of digestive enzymes and forming indigestible chemical complexes. These additives may be injected into meat, increasing the water content and thus the weight while drastically reducing nutritive value. If you buy frozen or ready-prepared meat products, these chemicals may be present in your food even when they are not specifically named on the label.

Many other chemicals in our food can act as anti-nutrients. Pesticide residues may reduce zinc absorption; one villain, 6-chloro-picalinic acid, is often used in crop growing.

The chemical contamination of food is a field full of unknowns. The many hazards of pesticides are only slowly being discovered; each one is said to be tested and safe when it's developed but experience and further research uncovers a host of unsuspected hazards. One after another, chemicals that were widely used and believed to be safe have been withdrawn (in developed countries, at least) because they are too dangerous. On top of this, different chemicals may interact with each other, and some change during cooking, processing or storage; there's virtually no information on these aspects of the problem. Then, to make matters worse, there are few effective controls over pesticide use even in this country, let alone in the third world countries from which we buy food.

Regrettably, there is far more incentive for industry to develop and use more and more of these chemicals than to investigate their potential dangers. Many food chemicals, particularly flavourings, are barely tested at all and only the manufacturer ever knows what they are; the products of their breakdown in cooking and storage, and their interaction with digestive enzymes, are unknown.

My attitude is that we don't need chemicals in our food and we're better off without them. Avoid them by eating organically grown food. If you cannot 'eat organic' all the time, at least avoid the most heavily contaminated foods where poisons are concentrated—organ meats such as liver, kidney and heart, and all animal fats.

When you eat organic, you will eat very little processed food. This means that you will automatically cut your intake of sugar, a non-food with marked anti-nutrient properties. Do not be persuaded that the purity of sugar or its association with energy means it's beneficial: you have no need whatever for sugar and your hormone balance will improve if you avoid it.

Sugar provides calories while depleting your body of the nutrients necessary to turn them into energy. Sugar increases excretion of the essential mineral chromium, thus reducing your ability to tolerate sugar. In addition, every time you have sugar, your body will use up B-group vitamins to cope with it—vitamins that you need to prevent PMT and other symptoms of hormone imbalance. Sugar has been shown to reduce hormone transport around the body; this may explain why women whose diet includes a lot of sugar suffer more problems with menopausal hot flushes than those who avoid it.

Eating sugar increases the risk that you'll experience sugar cravings. A vicious cycle can develop when your sugar tolerance falls and your blood sugar level becomes unstable. This is particularly likely to happen when the level of progesterone in your body is high, during the second half of the menstrual cycle, and in pregnancy. Poor sugar tolerance creates a dramatic fall in blood sugar when you haven't eaten for some hours. This fall is exaggerated by sugar, which induces a rush of insulin which takes sugar out of the blood and moves it into fat cells. Coffee and sweet drinks may make you feel better for an hour or so, but they create a dangerous hypoglycaemic (low blood sugar) reaction later.

Women who suffer from this sort of blood sugar instability often have weight problems; they may deny themselves food because they're afraid of getting even fatter, but are unable to deal with the sugar cravings that result. The answer is to avoid sugar and sweeteners *completely* and eat frequent wholefood snacks (such as wholemeal sandwiches) before you get too hungry. You'll find that by eating wholefoods earlier and avoiding the desperation that leads you to eat sugar, you'll start to lose that excess weight and you will have less difficulty with your blood sugar.

Brown sugar, fructose and glucose (ordinary sugar is a combination of fructose and glucose) are sometimes promoted as healthy alternatives to white sugar. Under normal circumstances you are better off without them. Avoid all sugars except for those that occur naturally in whole fruit and other foods, which come complete with the vitamins and minerals you need to benefit from them.

Some anti-nutrients that are particularly common in our diet and environment interfere with the metabolism and transport of nutrients that are crucial for hormone balance such as essential fatty acids and vitamin B_6. Many women whose diets and lifestyles are apparently good find they need supplements of these nutrients, and I believe that anti-nutrients are responsible.

Many women benefit from taking extra essential fatty acids in the form of evening primrose oil. One major type of anti-nutrient may explain why they are necessary: trans fatty acids, found in many of the fats in our diet. Trans fatty acids have a different chemical structure from the cis fatty acids that our bodies need. These two types of fat compete in the body so that the cells take up useless trans fats instead of valuable cis fats.

Cis fatty acids are essential for healthy cell membranes and for the normal production of prostaglandins, which are an essential part of many systems including those concerned with the sensation of pain. Prostaglandins act like local, tissue-level hormones, regulating cell function. The balance of the different prostaglandins in our bodies depends on the type of fat we eat; fatty acids in meat, cow's milk and eggs are used to make one series of prostaglandins, while the prostaglandins that maintain the healthy function of our reproductive organs are made from unprocessed vegetable oils and fish oils.

When our bodies build cell membranes from cis fats, the cells are more sensitive to hormones, particularly progesterone. If our bodies contain too high a proportion of trans fats, we need more progesterone to get the same effect so we suffer symptoms of progesterone deficiency. The results can be PMT, breast and menstrual pain, as well as dry skin, allergies and increased vulnerability to heart disease. If you suffer from any of these symptoms or you've found that supplements of essential fatty acids such as evening primrose oil are helpful, you will benefit from cutting out trans fats and eating only unprocessed fats such as cold-pressed oils, nut or seed spreads, and soft margarines such as good-quality sunflower spreads which contain a high proportion of polyunsaturated fat.

Trans fatty acids are found in most cheap fats. Food manufacturers prefer them because they not only keep the product price down, but have better keeping qualities. To reduce your intake, avoid hard margarine and cooking fats, bakery goods such as cakes, biscuits and pies, and repeatedly-heated fats such as those used in deep frying. Eat fish more often and reduce your intake of meat, eggs and cheese. Commercial fried foods like chips, crisps and doughnuts will reduce the availability of essential fatty acids to your body and the direct result can be pain associated with your menstrual cycle.

Vitamin B_6 deficiency, which is also widespread, seems similarly to be due to the proliferation of specific anti-nutrients. The main problem appears to be caused by chemicals called *hydrazines*, which are becoming ubiquitous in our environment. They are found in rocket fuels which, as a result of space flights, are released into the atmosphere; in ripening and sprouting inhibitors sprayed on to food crops; and in industrial chemicals. Some drugs, including oral contraceptives, contain derivatives of hydrazines. Some food additives including tartrazine (E102) are metabolised to hydrazine.

Other substances which increase our need for vitamin B_6 include heated and processed vegetable oils—substances that also, as we've seen, interfere with essential fatty acid status. But even if we cut out foods of this type, we cannot avoid exposure to all the chemicals that damage vitamin B_6-dependent enzyme systems. Although many of these chemicals—PCBs (poly-chlorinated biphenols) and pesticides such as DDT—have now been banned, they remain widespread in our environment; the body fat of animals and of people everwhere is polluted with them. In fact, women secrete these poisons in such large quantities in breast milk, that many babies are getting well over the safe limit as defined by the World Health Organization. It's inevitable then that we will need extra vitamin B$_6$, but our diets contain less than in the past.

Pesticides can cause a variety of metabolic problems. These chemicals are acknowledged poisons, designed to kill. Most of us, fortunately, are not exposed to high enough concentrations to cause obvious or immediate harm, but low concentrations put an inescapable demand on our bodies' detoxification systems. To cope with this while keeping all our systems working optimally, we have to maintain higher levels of nutrient input.

Crucial nutrients which protect our bodies from poisons include proteins, especially the sulphur-rich proteins in egg yolk, nuts and seeds. Selenium, zinc, and vitamins A, C and E are also essential for our bodies' de-toxification systems. The more we're exposed to environmental pollution, the more of these nutrients we need.

Smoking, of course, is the most pervasive sort of voluntary internal pollution. While cigarettes are not known to produce direct effects on our hormone systems, they contribute to related problems ranging from infertility to osteoporosis. Smoking causes indirect damage to hormone balance by increasing your need for de-toxifying vitamins and minerals to cope with the 200-plus poisons in tobacco smoke, thus reducing their availablility for hormone synthesis. Vitamin C, in particular, is depleted by smoking; this vitamin is important for the production of hormones in the adrenal glands.

Smokers know that their habit damages their health. It is saddening that young women, more than any other group, are taking up smoking, and that women are more reluctant to give up. If you're a smoker, changing your lifestyle to achieve a better hormone balance could provide the emotional stability you need to cope with quitting.

It is often difficult to pinpoint precise points of interaction between particular substances and our hormone systems. The situation is not so simple that we can say 'smoking reduces your progesterone levels' or 'pesticides interfere with oestrogen metabolism'. In natural systems, many pathways have a variety of different functions, and every part of the system interacts with every other part. Transport systems that move hormones around the body are also involved in moving other substances such as drugs. The enzyme systems in the liver metabolize nutrients, hormones and toxins; the more strain these systems have to endure through hormone imbalance, pollutant stress, or inadequate nutrition, the more problems you are likely to experience.

Obviously, if the system is totally overloaded with synthetic substances, there is less capacity for natural processes on which our hormone balance depends. Artificial chemicals, moreover, can damage metabolic systems, causing lasting problems. When those synthetic substances are closely related to natural hormones, the problems are likely to be more serious and specific. Enzyme systems which exist naturally to cope with sex hormones become crucial when the body has to deal with synthetic hormones. Not surprisingly, liver problems which can develop through the use of the contraceptive pill can produce long term hormone imbalance.

Poor diet—due to inadequate nutrient intake, slimming diets or the inclusion of anti-nutrients in poor-quality food—exacerbate these problems. If your diet is already low in vitamins or minerals, the moment you are exposed to anti-nutrients which increase your need for them, your problems will be multiplied. To protect yourself from anti-nutrients, you have to maintain a high nutritional status.

The first step in preventative action is to identify the anti-nutrients that are particularly important for you. Are you a tea-drinker or a sugar addict? Do you regularly eat chips, biscuits and doughnuts? Resolve to change. Replace your everyday anti-nutrients with nutrients: you'll be delighted at the effects.

Is the air you breathe polluted with chemicals that add to your nutrient needs? Let your nose be your guide—and don't damage its sensitivity with air fresheners or cigarette smoke. One disturbingly common pollutant is the fumes from burning plastics: the smoke contains dioxins and other poisons. Never put any form of plastic on a fire.

When you've taken action on all these fronts, the final problem—your ability to absorb nutrients—may be solved. But if you are sensitive to particular foods, you'll need to deal with this because food allergy reduces your nutrient absorption too. See chapter eight for advice on what to do.

Dealing with anti-nutrients could be your key to natural hormone health. You may not be able to avoid them completely but now you know about the problem, you'll certainly be able to reduce the severity of its effects.

CHAPTER SIX
Active Energy

Physical activity should be a crucial part of your strategy for optimum hormone balance. If you eat according to the advice given in the last two chapters, and walk briskly or take vigorous exercise for an average of half an hour every day, you can expect the following benefits:

- Freedom from period pain
- Freedom from breast pain
- Improved mood
- Diminished menopausal symptoms
- Freedom from the risk of osteoporosis in old age
- Freedom from weight problems.

Physical activity changes hormone balance in both the short and the long term. These changes are complex and not yet fully understood but a succession of research studies have proved that regular moderate exercise has tremendous practical benefits for hormone-related problems including period pain and PMT. Active women have less difficulty with pregnancy and childbirth, fewer menopausal symptoms and less osteoporosis after the menopause. Whatever your age and whatever your problem, more exercise is likely to help.

Many women don't realize just how important it is to be physically active. Exercise keeps all your organs and tissues in a healthy state and your body will not function at its best without it. But we live in a sedentary culture where most women drive or ride everywhere instead of using their own energy to get around, and sport is a minority option. The most obvious effect of all this inactivity is that the majority of women are flabby and unfit, and weight is a perpetual worry for two-thirds of the British female population. Problems with hormones are less obvious but just as common—and the two are closely connected because they have the same causes.

The fat content of your body is crucially dependent upon your activity level, and your hormone balance in turn is linked with the amount of fat in your body. Most women feel that they are fatter than they should be, but rather than increase their activity level, they try to diet. In the long term, food restriction makes you miserable and malnourished; in the short term, slimming diets reduce your ability to cope with pollutants and posions in the environment. Slimming diets don't keep you slim: they make you put on fat more easily by reducing the metabolic rate. Hormone problems are an inevitable consequence of this situation; if you restrict food intake, you don't get enough nourishment; and when you go short of nutrients, your whole hormone balance goes awry.

Activity and diet go hand in hand. When you eat more of the right types of food, you have more energy so you enjoy being more active. As I have explained in detail in the book I wrote with Colin Johnson, *Eat Yourself Thin*, this is the only long-term strategy that keeps you both slim and healthy. A higher rate of activity coupled with more good food produces a higher metabolic rate and a stronger, healthier, and better-balanced body. As you use your muscles more, you burn off excess fat and your hormone balance improves; and if you're underweight, you'll put on shapely curves as your muscles fill out. So make exercise a priority in your life—you'll look and feel much better for it!

There are many reasons why regular activity enhances hormone health, but the simple truth is that activity is necessary to the health of the whole body, and you can't expect to make one system healthy unless you look after the whole.

Hormone production involves many organs of the body. To function properly, every cell of every organ needs a good supply of blood, which carries the oxygen and nutrients that provide the energy for every chemical reaction on which life depends. Exercise increases blood-flow and ensures that the blood contains the oxygen we need. The liver, which transforms food into the components of enzymes, hormones and nutrients we can use, as well as de-toxifying the poisons we encounter every day and breaking down excess hormones, is crucial to every aspect of metabolism; but good liver function requires regular activity.

The glands which produce hormones also work better when you're physically active; the adrenal glands, for example, are stimulated into higher levels of hormone production by exercise. In addition, physical activity changes the sensitivity of cells to the effects of hormones, so that our hormone systems work more efficiently.

Strenuous activity produces rapid changes in all our hormone levels; scientists believe these are due to a direct influence on the pituitary gland which controls all our hormone systems. Exercise increases secretion of testosterone, progesterone, oestradiol, prolactin, cortisol, growth hormone, adrenalin and nor-adrenalin; it decreases secretion of insulin while increasing the sensitivity of the cells to insulin. The metabolic changes throughout our bodies are so profound that it's inevitable that exercise can make us feel completely different, both mentally and physically.

These adaptations increase the more often you exercise and the longer you persist. Within limits, the more you do, the more you benefit. However, it is possible to push your body too hard and produce a new form of imbalance. To avoid this, you need to recognize the warning signs of overdoing it. Loss of periods is the signal that a woman is doing too much.

In their research on female hormones, scientists have focused mainly on oestrogen. They have discovered that physical training reduces the total quantity of free oestrogen in the body and alters the pathway by which the body breaks oestrogen down, producing an inactive metabolite which is different from the active metabolite that predominates in sedentary women. Both these processes have similar effects: they reduce the effects of oestrogen in the body.

Regular strenuous training—such as dancers and other dedicated athletes subject themselves to—can reduce oestrogen levels to such a low level that periods cease and women become vulnerable to oestrogen-deficiency problems. If their body fat stores diminish too much, athletes become vulnerable to some of the problems that can afflict post-menopausal women. Skinny dancers, in particular, suffer stress fractures; in their efforts to stay light, they distort their hormone profiles so severely that they damage themselves.

As with most aspects of human health, going to the extreme is dangerous and unnecessary. It's not true that a woman can't be too thin: if you let that happen, the hormone changes can cause permanent damage through loss of bone. You must heed the warning signal of loss of periods: while you continue to have periods, you are likely to stay well. It is foolish to exercise or under-eat to such a degree that your periods stop; it may temporarily improve athletic performance, but that's pointless if your bones start breaking. If you've reached menopause, you're probably mature enough to be more sensible about excessive exercise, so this won't be relevant!

Less severe levels of exercise which move us just a little way down that road are entirely beneficial. You and I are unlikely to work our bodies anywhere near as hard as dedicated athletes, and there's no need to try!

One hormone that tends to go up rather than down with exercise is progesterone; half an hour's strenuous exercise can raise the level of progesterone in the circulation by 40 per cent. In practice, this means that progesterone-deficiency symptoms of PMT can improve within minutes of doing a physical work-out.

Regular moderate exercise has been shown in numerous surveys to lead to decreased PMT, especially decreased breast tenderness, fluid retention and mood-related symptoms. Periods get shorter, lighter and less troublesome. My personal experience has fully confirmed these benefits. Other women have observed them too. For example, Paula Weideger in *Female Cycles* (page 92) writes: 'I have noticed that when I ride my bike regularly and rely on it for transportation, I have almost no symptoms associated with menstruation.'

Improved vitamin metabolism is one consequence of better liver function which contributes to beneficial changes in hormone balance. Exercise increases the body's ability to use vitamin B_6, in addition to allowing you to eat more nutrient-rich food without putting on extra fat.

How much exercise is enough for you to reap the benefits? This depends on your age and the condition of your body. Going for the burn, stressing yourself really hard so that you ache for days, or indeed going to any extreme, is neither necessary nor wise. To improve your hormone balance and your exercise capacity, you need to work within your current capacity; do as much as you can comfortably achieve on a regular basis, gradually increasing the amount you do as your body adapts. That way, you will experience only the improvements and avoid becoming disenchanted with exercise by damaging yourself.

The key concept is enjoyment. Go for the pleasure principle; take up activities you enjoy and do more of them.

The amount and type of exercise your body will benefit from varies with your age. Young women (25 and under) can work their bodies hard in vigorous sport. You will stay lean and, by keeping your oestrogen production in check, protect yourself from hormone-related cancers in later life. Rose Frisch of Harvard University has studied these effects in detail; she discovered that students who were athletic at university were much less likely to develop cancers of the breast, uterus, cervix and vagina when they grew older.

Regular hard games of tennis or squash are great for young women who want to be fit and lean. Wild dancing, running, hard cycling, gym training and other demanding forms of activity are excellent and fun. Work your body hard for half an hour three times a week, and you'll be doing yourself a lasting favour. If you want to do more than this, you'll come to no harm—so long as you keep on menstruating. But beware obsession: it is dangerous to ignore warning signals from your body. If you start to miss periods or go down with frequent infections, you are overdoing it. Make your training schedule a bit easier and rest for longer.

For women who are thinking about starting their families, a slightly lighter exercise schedule is best. Adult women should be plumper than adolescents; pregnancy will be easier and their babies will be stronger and healthier. However, most women in their mid-twenties are already growing too fat because they aren't sufficiently active; a moderate level of exercise will make you feel and look better.

Between the ages of perhaps twenty and thirty-five—the years when you're most likely to consider pregnancy—a schedule of mixed activities is best. Alternate between long, easy activities like long walks and cycle rides, and shorter periods of vigorous activity. You might play tennis or dance twice a week and go for a five-mile walk twice a week; or get your bike roadworthy and cycle everywhere, sometimes fast and hard, sometimes more gently, depending on how you feel. That way, you'll continue to look the way you did at twenty for another two or three decades. Your face may change a bit but your body won't sag or lose its youthful definition, and your periods won't bother you at all.

For the women who's getting closer to menopause—roughly

between 35 and 50—it's best to concentrate on activites that are moderately demanding but not too strenuous. You don't want to get thin; your priority is to maintain and build your strength, to keep a high level of lean muscle bulk, and to develop strong bones that will stay intact through the menopause and into old age.

As we grow older, we become more vulnerable to strain and damage, and our bodies mend less quickly. Our activities should take account of this. Older women will benefit from some quite heavy activities but only when they are strong enough to cope with them. Building up this strength gradually and steadily is the key. Regularly graded work-outs with instruction in a gym will achieve progressive increments in muscle power and strength which will make you look and feel younger and fitter.

Whatever type of activity you choose, it's wise to build on a solid bed rock of overall fitness. The best way to create this is through walking; nothing is more beneficial for women's health than regular long walks.

Women are designed for walking. Our legs are very strong in relation to the rest of our body, and our muscle fuelling systems are uniquely adapted to steady, long-lasting exercise. Women have relatively more fat than men, and less glycogen (the body's short-term energy store); and the female enzyme systems are biased towards the use of fat as fuel. The types of exercise that burn fat predominantly are not very demanding, but they can and should be continued for a long time. The male body, with its large muscles and glycogen reservoirs, is better constructed for rapid, intensive work, while the female metabolism is better suited to the use of fat for extended activity. The longer you walk, the more fat your muscles will burn.

Walking is particularly important for the health of older women. Menopausal and post-menopausal women (aged fifty and over) are particularly vulnerable to osteoporosis, which causes weak bones which fracture easily. Chapter 10 explains fully how to prevent osteoporosis, but walking is a vital part of the strategy. Women who walk regularly are much less likely to suffer bone fractures.

Some elderly women are anxious about tripping over and breaking limbs when they go walking. But you're much more likely to fall on a frosty morning when you dash out to the corner shop, or trip over a carpet at home, than to fall on your walk providing you're wearing the right kind of shoes. Since you can't avoid the risk of falling over, you should act to prevent serious damage from any fall. And that means keeping your muscles and bones strong by regular walking.

The longer you spend walking, the healthier your bones will be. It's virtually impossible to walk too much but it's very easy to walk too little in our urban society. In addition, regular walking will keep your weight down, minimize arthritis, reduce your risk of heart and circulatory disease, and keep your skin healthy—it's great all-round exercise.

So whether you're sixteen or sixty, get your walking shoes on and get out there in the fresh air! Always hold your head up proudly, keep your back straight and your pelvis flexible, and walk from the hip. Walk briskly and determinedly, swinging your arms and breathing deeply. Wear comfortable shoes— middle-range trainers, designed for runners, are best—and cotton or wool socks to keep your feet fresh. Choose loose clothes which won't constrict your breathing or circulation and remove layers as you warm up.

Walk the tension out of your system, walk that excess fat off your tummy, walk the pain out of your periods! Walk all the paths in your area, explore and discover the hidden places that you can't find in any other way. Walk the local canal tow path, the woods and disused railway lines; walk along rivers, over hills, through parts and around fields. Avoid major roads where the air is polluted with traffic fumes; choose quiet byways and leafy suburbs. London is a delightful walking city; you can get right away from the traffic, into the parks and wild spaces.

Pick your routes with the help of a good large-scale map or walking guide. If you're worried about muggers or rapists, remember that the chance of encountering such people is much, much less than the risk of breaking your hip as a result of your bones being weak. Of course, you wouldn't choose to walk in the more violent areas of our cities. The risk of violence is regrettably exaggerated by the media which thrive on horror stories while ignoring everyday disasters that don't make the news.

When you walk in cities, especially at night, protect yourself with confident body-language. Research has shown that attackers do not go for people who stand straight and show no sign of fear in their posture. So when you're walking the correct way, the way that will prevent aches and make your walk feel good, you are also looking after your personal safety. Any walker will tell you: you don't get threatened when you walk with confidence. If you're still nervous, go out with friends or dogs; form a walking group with your neighbours. You'll soon discover that you have nothing to fear.

Walking takes a little time, but health is your most valuable asset and if you don't devote time to looking after yourself, you sacrifice your health. There's no sense in short term planning or convenience that causes possibly irreversible long term damage. It takes far less time than the average woman spends slumped in front of the TV, and you'll discover that your walking time is actually far more relaxing than the mindless lounging that we regard as relaxation. When you walk regularly, you'll relax more profoundly and sleep more deeply. Make it a lifetime priority and plan time for walking into your week.

If you think 'walkies!' every day, you'll find plenty of opportunities to get out there and exercise your legs. Many women invariably get into their cars to go shopping, even if shops are less than half a mile away. It's a question of attitudes and assumptions: but because your health is valuable, you should avoid using the car whenever possible.

Think about the ways you can enhance the pleasure of walking. Get a personal stereo if listening to music encourages you to walk further; or take a dog—your neighbour's dog if you don't have one of your own. Elderly dog-owners often appreciate friendly dog-walkers. If you're sociable and enjoy planned walks, join your local rambler's group; the contact numbers will be in the library.

To sum up, do anything you can to get yourself outside and walking! Don't make excuses like 'I'm on my feet all day'—that's not the same at all; you need to walk to help your legs and feet cope with the demand of standing too long. Walk all day if you can; walk for ten minutes whenever you can. You can't do too much.

Cycling is almost as health-giving as walking and you may prefer it. It's great for everyone. Go to that bike-obsessed country, the Netherlands, and you'll see people of all ages, from tiny tots to old ladies in traditional dress, on their bikes.

Cycling is one of the best exercises for period pain. Cycle hard in the days before you expect your period, and you'll suffer far less. Cycle when the pain comes on, and you could find it disappears completely. I recall one day (before I understood the nature of the problem sufficiently to avoid the pain) when I was on my bike all morning—when I got off, I'd be doubled up so I just got back on again! By afternoon the pain had gone and I was feeling much better for my hours in the saddle. The advantage of cycling is that there's less jarring to the pelvis than when you're walking, yet there's constant leg movement to keep the pelvic muscles and circulation working. You may imagine that activity is the last thing you want when your belly's sore but you'll be pleasantly surprised if you just drop your assumptions and get on your bike.

You don't have a bike or you can't ride? It's never too late! I was well into my thirties before I started. Sometimes I felt a bit foolish, learning with my four-year-old neighbour who got her first bike at the same time, but I did learn eventually and I've found cycling tremendously liberating and a source of unexpected joy. I go cycling when I don't feel energetic because it gives me energy; I cycle when I'm feeling down because the wind in my hair lifts my spirits. I cycle for pleasure and because cycling is a non-polluting form of transport; I cycle in central London because it's the most efficient way to get around. I just wish there were more cyclists so our needs would be taken seriously by road-builders.

When you're cycling, wear bright, reflective clothing and study maps to find quiet routes. Get a bike that suits you and make sure it's correctly adjusted. A comfortable saddle is essential; go to a specialist bike shop and get a ladies' touring saddle that feels good under your bum. And then get out there and ride! You'll feel much better for it.

Aerobics and dance can be good for everyone too, but if you join a class, be sure it's right for your level of fitness. There's no point struggling to keep up with a bunch of exercise freaks and feeling sore and foolish at the end of it. The crucial point about exercise is you need to enjoy it enough to carry on doing it—not just next week or next month, but next year and for the rest of your life. So if it doesn't feel right, don't push yourself; just carry on trying different activities until you find one that you enjoy.

Dance is wonderful for self-expression and emotional catharsis. You can throw your feelings into it, getting carried away by music and movement. If you're self-conscious (most of us are!), try dancing alone to your favourite records. Don't feel restricted to what is generally thought of as dancing music; you can dance to Beethoven quartets if you're in the mood!

In your dance, reach and twist and bend in every way you can. Use your whole body, keeping the rhythm going with your feet.

Jump and run across the room, let yourself go! Forget dance steps, you are creating your own dance, the dance that matches your own feelings and personality.

Even the bed-ridden can dance in their own way. If you're in a wheelchair, you can still dance with those parts of your body that retain mobility. Dance is different for every person. It has no limits.

Aerobics and floor exercises are more structured and often directed at working particular sets of muscles for particular reasons. The danger with this is that you can over-do it quite easily if you're doing an unfamiliar routine. Sore muscles don't help anyone. Stop before the pain starts and forget about 'going for the burn'. Frankly, it's stupid. Going for the burn is more likely to give you strained muscles and ligaments with the result that you give it all up, than to create a figure like Jane Fonda's.

I like the Canadian Airforce routine shown in *Physical Fitness* (Penguin). If you follow the instructions, you won't strain yourself but you will gradually increase your level of fitness with a balanced routine. Sometimes I do exercises and then dance for a while; sometimes I resent the constraints of formal exercise routines so I just dance. Other times, when I'm going for ruthless efficiency, I do exercises only. Follow your moods; do what fits at the time but do it! You'll be healthy only if you're active.

Swimming is the exercise that tops the popularity polls in surveys among women, but how many actually do it? When did you last swim? (When did I last swim, come to that?) It's great if you do it, and it's especially beneficial if you're not very fit or supple and you need exercise that won't put too much strain on your legs. However, it does have one disadvantage for mature women and those of us who use exercise to prevent future bone problems: it doesn't significantly increase bone density because the water takes your body weight. If you like swimming, do something else as well, like walking. That way, you enjoy all the benefits.

Running is marvellous for cardiovascular fitness and for weight loss. It has some disadvantages, however. First, you have to be quite fit to run; running produces dramatic changes in the body because it is demanding. You have to be well motivated and persistent; start gently and practise regularly, extending the distance you cover and increasing your speed gradually.

If you do decide to run, you will in due course experience pleasures that match the effort you put into it. Regular runners enjoy a 'runner's high' which is one effect of the stress that running puts on your body. This type of stress produces a surge of the brain's natural opiate hormones which induce profound happiness, reduce pain, and speed up healing. The more often you run, the quicker you'll experience this phenomenon. Regular runners can become addicted to it, feeling flat and depressed when they're not able to run.

Running is hard work. You'll benefit in proportion to the work that you put into it, but you have to be aware of the limitations of your body. When you're unwell, you must not run. If you feel a cold or infection coming on, you must not run. If you're suffering aches or strains in your legs, you must take it easy because you can damage yourself. Err on the side of caution then return to running gently as soon as you can.

I use running to shed excess fat quickly after a period of inactivity (sitting at a word processor is definitely bad for the figure!) or when I feel my naturally plump self would not be a good advertisement for some of my books. When I haven't run for a long time, it can be difficult to get started; but when I get into the habit of running again, it makes me feel great. My skin glows, my hair shines and my tummy shrinks.

Surveys show that running is very good for your mood. Between 60 and 92 per cent of female runners report psychological benefits: an improved sense of well-being, reduced anxiety and tension, enhanced self-image and confidence. 69 per cent of women report that running reduces depression. In general, athletes are less anxious, depressed, tense, angry, confused and tired than non-athletes. For my part, I know that if I can get out running when I'm sliding into despair for any reason, the mood will often disappear completely so that by the time I've cooled down and washed the sweat off, I feel serene and able to cope.

If you're thinking about starting, build up your fitness first with long, brisk walks. Alternate walking and trotting, going faster at intervals till you're tired and then going slower while you recover. As you get fitter, you'll be able to run more until you're running miles at a stretch. Don't bother to train for marathons unless you really want that sense of achievement; recreational running is better for your health than the heavy demand of marathon training.

Ideally, women should aim to run between 10 and 20 miles a week in three sessions. While you're out, vary your pace; don't jog interminably at one speed: sprint sometimes and walk at others. You'll use a larger range of muscles and enjoy greater benefits.

Running is especially suitable for the under-fifties. If you're in your twenties or thirties and starting to spread around the middle, take up running—it'll help you keep your youth. If you're still running at menopause, you're very unlikely to suffer from hot flushes because your temperature control will be much better tuned by the regular production of internal heat alternating with cooling. But women of this age should beware of running so much or eating so little that they get thin; that could reduce oestrogen production too fast and cause unnecessary problems.

For younger age-groups, speed is exciting and beneficial. Fast racquet games like squash are perfect for women in their teens and twenties; older women will do better with tennis, while badminton is the best game for middle-aged and elderly women because it doesn't put so much strain on the upper body.

Play an active game and keep it going as long as you can. Singles matches are generally better than doubles because you keep moving. Play with your partner, your friends or your children—racquet games are fun for everybody!

There are many health-giving sports I haven't mentioned here, from rowing to cross-country skiing. Whatever form of exercise you choose, your general health will benefit and any hormone problems will decrease. If you suffer from diabetes or hypo-glycaemia, problems which are particularly acute when your hormone balance goes awry in the second half of the menstrual cycle, activity is crucial to reduce your insulin requirements and keep your blood sugar stable.

Exercise is the key to active management of your hormones. If you want to go beyond hormone health to deliberate control of your physiological balance, you can vary your activity level and the types of activity you choose to move towards creating a body that matches your particular needs. You can make yourself more 'masculine' by adopting an exercise pattern more characteristic of the male, or more 'female' by choosing feminine patterns of exercise.

Masculine activities are those that make heavy demands on your body, and which cannot be sustained for long periods: anaerobic, rather than aerobic exercise. Running, weight training and downhill skiing are examples: they are very strenuous and they make you pant heavily. If you push yourself to your personal limits in activities of this kind you will notice immediate changes in your physiological balance which will be quickly reflected in your body shape and composition. I use activities like these to raise my metabolic rate, to get thinner and to develop my physical strength. Healthy men are naturally more muscular and leaner than women and the more our activities mirror their more thrusting, powerful, goal-directed approach, the more our bodies adapt by moving towards the male pattern.

Predictably, these changes are mediated by a change in hormone balance. I find that when I push myself in the masculine direction for a few weeks, I'm more likely to grow hairs on my face—but I'm more assertive and sexier too, for these aspects of behaviour are stronger when male hormone levels are higher.

If you feel your problems are linked with a body or behaviour that tends too much towards the soft and feminine, you might do well to adopt these aspects of the male lifestyle. Conversely, women who are rather masculine in build, naturally lean (though maybe with a tendency to a thick waistline) and perhaps more thrusting in their approach to life, can move towards the shapely female with more feminine patterns of exercise. Sustained and relaxing activities such as walking, to which the female is so well adapted, help to rebalance female hormones.

Naturally, changes such as these need to be underpinned with appropriate dietary modification. If you're putting the heavy demands on your body that the masculinizing approach involves, you have to eat relatively larger meals, with plenty of protein. I find that it works better if I eat more fish and eggs and slightly less carbohydrate. But if you want to move towards the feminine, you should nibble; have many smaller, high-carbohydrate meals and snacks to sustain the long-lasting female pattern of energy output. Whatever activity pattern you choose, you must have enough nutritious food to keep you going and maintain your energy levels. You just won't feel able to do as much as you intend if you don't get enough nourishment.

Improving your personal health and achieving the right balance in your own life is only part of the reason for increasing your activity level. The other part is to encourage your children to be active. Your example is crucial; if you don't exercise, your children aren't likely to exercise either. And when they grow up, they'll probably suffer worse imbalance and worse health than you do. Women are responsible for the health of the next generation; it is a responsibility that most take very seriously but few understand completely.

The developing health problems in our daughters are serious; the present generation of children are the fattest and least fit of any previous generation. This is no coincidence when mothers habitually drive their offspring to schools to which everyone used to walk; when the chief pastimes are watching TV and videos, not active games; when labour-saving devices have taken the effort out of virtually every household task. Health educators are sounding warnings about the threat of cardiovascular disease when today's children reach adulthood; but the circulation is just one of the body systems that requires physical activity for healthy function.

When a fat, inactive girl grows up, she is immediately a candidate for serious hormone imbalance. PMT will develop earlier for her than for her active sister; periods will start sooner, be heavier and more troublesome. Research has shown that the children of active mothers are in turn more active; they follow their parents' lead. If you have children, you owe it to them to be physically active and to exercise regularly. That's the only way you can encourage them to do the same.

Through regular activity, you will safeguard your own future and your children's future. If you haven't seriously considered regular exercise or sport, think deeply about it now. You owe it to yourself and to your family to prevent not only short-term miseries of hormone imbalance but also its long-term consequences—breast cancer and osteoporosis.

So, get out there—get moving! It's good for you and it's fun!

CHAPTER SEVEN
The Female Mind and the Female Body

Everything that affects the body also affects the mind; hormone changes are no exception to this rule. Conversely, our thoughts and emotions have a profound influence on our hormone balance and its effects on our bodies. We cannot separate mental, physical, emotional, spiritual and social aspects of ourselves; this is the central idea of the holistic approach to health.

When any change in one part of our lives produces changes in all the others, we get a distorted picture of what's going on if we only deal with selected aspects in isolation. Western medicine and science concentrates on physical phenomena, which are relatively easily to measure, manipulate, and assess. The scientific approach works with tiny, carefully defined aspects of life, looking for specific effects which can be easily and reliably recorded. Consequently, medicine exaggerates the importance of physical things while denying the relevance of the more intangible. If doctors are unable to pin our experience of pain or distress to obvious physiological malfunction, they may dismiss it as imaginary or unimportant.

For many years, most doctors asserted that women's problems with periods, menopause, and other aspects of hormone balance were due to our refusal to accept our role in society. Women's illnesses (along with some other conditions which science could not explain, like asthma) were seen as psychological in origin and women who suffered in these ways were dismissed as hysterical misfits. Millions were given tranquillizers to calm them down while real problems were left untreated.

Today the pendulum is swinging the other way. Emotional distress is sometimes seen entirely as a manifestation of biochemical imbalance. Scientists search for clear-cut links between hormone levels and mental state, hoping to explain depression or tension in terms of abnormal levels of hormones. Most have failed: for example, Dr David Rubinow and his colleagues at the National Institute of Mental Health in Maryland, could find no difference in hormone levels between women who suffered pre-menstrual mood changes and those who did not.

Nevertheless, some doctors assert that fluctuating hormone levels have straightforward effects on the brain. Dr Guy Abraham, a specialist in the nutritional links of pre-menstrual syndrome, believes that progesterone is a generalized central nervous system depressant which causes depression, while high oestrogen levels cause tension and anxiety. Unfortunately, this simple picture doesn't actually fit women's experience.

To begin with, we frequently experience tension and depression together. If it were a simple matter of too much of one hormone or too much of another, we'd suffer one state or the other, not both. Dr Abraham's own research reveals that most women have both problems and only a tiny majority have clearcut anxiety without depression, or depression without anxiety. Our reactions to changing hormone levels are individual and variable.

This variability results partly from the way we react to the changes in our bodies, and our perception of their significance. What we feel depends on the way we interpret different body states and the meaning we give to them. At the same time, our mental processes affect our bodies and can affect hormone-related changes.

The parts of the brain that are involved in thought, memory and sensation are connected by direct neural pathways with emotional centres, and then with the pituitary gland which controls hormone output. The pituitary is actually suspended from the hypothalamus, which controls emotion, appetite and desire. Neurochemists have isolated substances produced by the hypthalamus which act on the pituitary. These are neuro-hormones, direct parallels of the hormones produced by the pituitary which then control the total balance of hormones in the body. The whole body is thus controlled and modulated by input from the brain.

At the same time, the brain responds to chemical changes within the body, adjusting feelings and thought to take account of physical change. Psychologists have demonstrated that we can react in a whole variety of ways to a single hormone stimulus, depending on the context and our expectations. How we feel, how we react and what we imagine to be happening to us, is subject to mental modification. For example, people injected with the stress/alertness hormone adrenalin will feel angry and get aggressive when confronted with an irritating experimenter but laugh and have a very good time with a joky experimenter. Either way, their reactions are exaggerated by the hormone; but the specific reaction they experience cannot be predicted by biochemistry alone.

To complicate the picture further, sex hormones alter the metabolism of the chemicals that make our nerves work. Within the nervous system, each nerve fires when a minute electric current passes along it. At the end of the nerve, where it connects to other nerves, there is a bulge containing microscopic quantities of neurotransmitters, specialized chemicals that can jump across the gap (called the synapse) between one nerve and the next, setting up an electric potential that makes the second nerve fire.

In the brain, each of these synaptic junctions has many connections, each with a different balance of neurotransmitters. The outgoing nerve will react in different ways to different quantities and mixtures of neurotransmitters. Some transmitters amplify the effects of others and increase the electrical activity in certain parts of the brain, while others are inhibitory. A single transmitter will be inhibitory under some circumstances and excitatory under others. Activity in one part of the brain will reduce the reactivity in some other parts, while increasing reactivity in others.

It is thus very difficult to relate mood, behaviour or hormone change to fluctuations in the levels of neurotransmitters. Neurochemists have worked out some general principles but they are crude in comparison with the intricacy of the brain itself.

Oestrogen is believed to alter the rate of breakdown of neurotransmitters. If a particular transmitter breaks down rapidly, its level in the brain will tend to fall, whereas when breakdown is slow, it will rise. The substances that break down neurotransmitters are called monoamine oxidases (MAOs), and there are many different kinds which react with each of the transmitters. To complicate matters further, oestrogen affects different MAOs to different degrees.

Scientists seem to argue that high oestrogen levels lead to increased breakdown of dopamine, the transmitter that's particularly important for precise control of movement. Changes in dopamine transmission in the brain is likely to affect mood, too, but we understand too small a part of this complex picture to make precise predictions about the effects produced.

Oestrogen is said to produce a relative excess of serotonin and nor-adrenalin, transmitters which are important for sleep and alertness. But many brain structures have serotonin and nor-adrenalin working in opposition. So while we can assume that changing oestrogen levels will affect the brain, we can't judge from the neurochemistry what these effects might be. Add in the effects of the other hormones, and the picture becomes impossibly complicated.

We can anticipate subtle mental changes of many kinds but not their precise nature. Every aspect of brain function will be affected, the sensitivity of our senses and the intensity of our feelings, the memories we recall and the sharpness of our wit, the precision of our movements and the expression of our desires. Hormone balance is likely to affect the ease with which we fall asleep and our energy when awake. Every single aspect of life is affected by hormone fluctuations.

Does this mean that we are really victims of our hormones, 'nought but a jangle of hormones', as my partner used to say I was? The answer is both yes and no. If things get seriously out of balance, you will be at the mercy of uncontrollable impulses and instability. But while you keep yourself in balance, sweet reason (or passion, or patience) can prevail.

If you've suffered from the mental distortion that severe hormone imbalance such as uncontrolled PMT creates, you'll be familiar with hormone-induced insanity. I ceased to be sane when I took oral contraceptives; some brands made me clinically depressed and incapable of thinking or keeping up with my work so I had to have a year off university; others made me so abnormally aggressive and paranoid that my partner saw I'd gone crazy and took the pills away from me, upon which I emerged as from a dreadful dream.

When your brain is thrown badly out of balance by an unsuitable hormone state, everything can go out of control. Under normal circumstances most of us can avoid this sort of situation, although it has been demonstrated that women with diagnosed mental illness are most likely to be admitted to hospital during the pre-menstrual period. For these women, as for me when I took the contraceptive pill, the edge of insanity is so close that quite a small increment in imbalance can tip them off. Learning to maintain a healthy balance is especially important for such vulnerable women.

Hormones are just one class of substances that affects brain transmitter systems. The food you eat, the chemicals you absorb, and your micro-nutrient status can affect your mind both directly and indirectly. Everything that affects your brain has overall consequences for the body systems that are controlled by the brain.

Similarly, if your body is subjected to stress of any sort, brain hormone levels change as the brain co-ordinates its systems for coping. For example, if you exercise until you're exhausted, the levels of nor-adrenaline and other neurotransmitters rise. This is what produces the increased sense of relaxed alertness that follows intense activity; and many people swim or run in the mornings before work in order to induce this mental change.

Brain hormones, sex hormones, and the other hormones all work together in harmony. Regular exercise, a balanced diet and adequate rest will help keep all of them at their optimum levels. You will notice benefits both in your physical functioning and your mental state.

This means that we can work on hormone-related problems in a variety of ways that take advantage of the interlinkage between mind and body. We can work on improving our physical health and enjoy mental benefits; at the same time, if we resolve our emotional problems, we will enjoy better physical functioning. And when we tune our minds into what we are doing with our bodies, all the benefits will be enhanced.

In general, the brain seems to aim for consistency. Experience has to have meaning—even if we have to seek out the meaning by interpreting something in an unusual way. You're probably familiar with feeling irritable and quickly finding something to get irritated about so that the internal sensation makes sense. I used to experience this situation every month for a few days before my period. Part of my mind would often be coolly aware that I was picking on my partner because of what was going on within myself, rather than what he was doing; but my mind would quickly adjust to allow me to ignore unwelcome wisdom and focus on his monstrous behaviour! If, instead of ignoring reality, I'd achieved consistency by accepting my hyper-sensitive state and dealt with that by eating and going for a calming walk, we should have avoided considerable conflict. Perhaps, though,

I needed to express that anger and hadn't been able to get it out of my system.

Most women are well aware of the way hormone-related problems vary with emotional state. If I'm going through a bad patch with my partner, fighting, feeling rejected or under-appreciated, I'm much more likely to suffer pre-menstrual physical symptoms like water retention. Domestic upheavals or unhappiness at work can precipitate menstrual problems. It's not unusual to cease ovulating and miss periods when you're under emotional strain; in students, the regular cycle can disappear completely during the first stressful terms away from home, or when exams begin. Some women have infertility problems during periods of mental stress; when it's over, they are able to get pregnant.

So if you are under mental strain, you should not be surprised if your hormones go awry. Work done on resolving the conflicts in your life may also solve your hormone problems.

Our bodies function normally when life as a whole is running smoothly, without causing us undue excessive stress. We can't expect life to be like this all the time—it would be boring if it were! But when we have hormone problems, we should aim to move towards a way of life that's balanced at all levels. It's foolish to concentrate solely on making physical adjustments if your greatest problems are emotional; your time might be better spent talking to a counsellor than going to the gym.

Fluctuations in mental state that accompany hormone changes affect the way we deal with emotional issues. One fascinating study of memory and the menstrual cycle revealed that women recall happy events more readily around ovulation and unpleasant events in the pre-menstrual period. You may feel deeply resentful towards your partner because of what you perceive as past wrongs but if you can only recall the reasons for your anger when you're pre-menstrual, you aren't likely to do that particular emotional work at any other time. It may seem unpleasant but if you take advantage of this hormonal spur to memory, you may be able to resolve those problems through discussion.

I have come to see a healthy balance between the accepting state of early-to-mid-month and the more critical state that stretches from post-ovulation to the second day or so of my period. I'm not totally one person or the other, and though it might seem preferable to be sunny and uncritical all the time, my needs would get ignored and I'd become everybody's dogsbody instead of my own person. Better by far that I stand and fight for balanced relationships when my internal state is right, even if I don't seem such a nice person; but, now I keep myself in a better physical balance, the fights no longer go out of control.

When we're distressed, that pre-menstrual negativism which can be valuable in the right balance, may become excessive and tip our delicate equilibrium out of balance. A feedback cycle develops where you feel bad about the world and yourself, neglect yourself, then feel worse. Hormone imbalances and physical symptoms may make you feel physically sick as well as mentally sore. At this point you have to retire from conflict, rest and look after yourself. Isolating yourself with a good book in bed sometimes seems the best thing of all by the time the period starts after stormy pre-menstrual days! Your excuse may be that you're nursing a sore tummy but the truth is that you're doing a lot more—acting to meet your own personal needs in your own way.

Sometimes, pre-menstrual mental changes can be very positive. Instead of anger, you may experience a surge of energy and creativity. It is regrettable that because of the predominance of negative experiences and views of the pre-menstrual days, this facet of hormone-related mood change has tended to be ignored. Researchers have concentrated on the anxious and depressed women rather than the minority who enjoy enhanced well-being. In addition, women who are asked to recall pre-menstrual experience are more likely to report negative aspects than those who are questioned during the pre-menstrual phase. This has produced a consistent bias in research results which can influence our interpretation of what happens to us, making us feel worse than we need.

While our mental state certainly changes with our hormone cycles, our experience reflects the interaction of these changes with life circumstances. Unhappy women may interpret non-specific arousal as tension while happy women interpret it as increased vigour. Emotional arousal fuels a fight when your partnership is under strain, and intensifies excitement when you're in love.

Cyclical changes can be found in every aspect of behaviour. Thinking, feeling, memory, sexual interest and responsiveness are just some of the variables that have been linked with hormone change.

One would expect that sex should be more appealing when we're at our most fertile, around ovulation. For some women, this is unquestionably the case; there's a clear peak in sexual activity at mid-month. I've often observed this in myself: I'm at my randiest just before and during the day I ovulate. Since my mid-twenties, I've been aware of ovulation, which causes a distinctive near-painful sensation on alternating sides of my lower abdomen, and I've come to associate that sensation with a sometimes overwhelming lust. In fact, so strong is the influence of my hormones that I at one point took to warning men of my fickleness if an affair began at this time; I'd found so often that I was only interested in them sexually during these few days! Not that any man took the warning seriously: nobody said, OK, let's wait a week and see how we feel...

Mid-month is the time for the most memorable candlelit dinners. You'll be at your most attractive, your skin glowing, your conversation up-beat. If only all our important appointments fell on the right days!

Had any potential lover decided to heed my warnings about fickleness and waited a week, he'd have found me at my sexual lowest. In this too, I am not atypical. For a few days I am simply not interested in sex. I may feel affectionate but not sexual. And if I do get involved in sexual activity, it doesn't mean a lot or do a lot for me: some essential part just isn't switched on. Other women have described this phenomenon and surveys show that sexual interest does indeed fall rapidly a day after ovulation to reach a trough around the end of the third week of the cycle.

During the fourth week, despite our tendency to be irritable, sexual interest often rises again. This is the time for me when sex can be comforting. Women are most likely to masturbate and quite likely to initiate sexual activity with partners just before their periods.

A couple of days into the period, there's another peak of sexual responsiveness and interest. For some women this is the best time, but we have to come to terms with menstrual taboos and cope with the messiness of intercourse and that's enough to put many people off. In addition, women who use tampons suffer from vaginal dryness because tampons don't just soak up blood but also vaginal secretions; in fact, sometimes the drying is so severe that the vagina becomes sore and ulcerated. So practicalities may interfere with feeling, distorting our sexual behaviour.

Many cultures have sexual taboos around menstruation. Moslems and Jews are two religious groups for whom sex during the period is forbidden. This is very frustrating for those women whose sex drive is heightened at this time.

Some psychologists believe that women are more sensitive to strong stimuli during the pre-menstrual days. We react more violently to what's going on around us. We respond more strongly to social stimuli too, noticing other people's behaviour more readily, so we'll feel more readily slighted if we're already feeling negative about ourselves.

I used to be very difficult to live with at these times. Depression stood close behind my shoulder. Rage would build up at the slightest provocation: I'd flash hot, disintegrated, even murderous and I'd feel I could fight to the death, because I didn't give a damn about death.

Violent crimes can be committed by women who are in this state. Judges may let women off to seek treatment, but it's no victory if we are classified as crazy for a substantial part of our lives. We need to understand and conquer the craziness, understand our vulnerability and prevent over-reaction by looking after our needs so that we don't topple into such crises of hormone-induced mental imbalance. We can hold on to the adult part of ourselves, keeping the child with her unfettered impulses under control, if we acknowledge our instability and take action to deal with it sensibly. The mind-set that can keep us on an even keel permits us to admit we're vulnerable, but recognizes that we can act to reduce that vulnerability. Sometimes we have to withdraw to attend to our personal needs, putting problems aside until we feel stronger.

Although we may easily get distraught and feel we can't cope, women are often able to think faster in this state of pre-menstrual arousal. Reaction times and the ability to do mental arithmetic have been shown to be quicker. However, the performance of women who suffer from pre-menstrual distress is, as one would anticipate, very variable when they're doing difficult or complex tasks.

Although we may be capable of reacting faster, road accidents are in fact more common in the days before the period. Driving is certainly a complex task and when your performance is unreliable, you may not drive safely. I have observed that I forget important moves like checking all my mirrors before changing lanes in traffic. It's useful to get to know your own reactions so that you can allow for them; if you drive in a highly-stressed state of mind, your judgement may be poor. For a while, when I suffered badly from this problem, I would refuse to drive during the few critical days of my period: it was too risky.

We should not assume, though, that we're generally less competent in the second half of the month. We're just *different*. Earlier in the month, we're more easily distracted and we concentrate less well. Studies have shown that women complete IQ tests faster but with less accuracy before ovulation, more slowly and more accurately during the pre-menstrual week.

The way we interpret menstrual changes is important for the way we feel when they happen. If you can't stand the sight or smell of menstrual blood, or you feel bad about being female, you're more likely to be tense and to experience menstruation as painful. So making the best of your period means accepting your female nature. Accustom yourself to the changes in vaginal discharges; get used to the smells and textures. You could try smelling or tasting the blood—you'll discover it's not repulsive at all!

Hormone-related mental and emotional changes are not restricted to the cyclic fluctuations of the menstrual cycle. During pregnancy, when sex hormone levels rise higher than at any other time in a woman's life, moods and feelings form a unique pattern. Many women feel quite placid during late pregnancy; there's often a sense of acceptance, of quietness, possibly because of the staggeringly high progesterone output at this time. But if the social context makes the woman anxious about becoming a mother, this quietness could be experienced as depression.

After the birth, progesterone and other sex hormones fall precipitously and this is a time when women become particularly vulnerable to all forms of mental illness. Post-natal depression may be due to these hormone changes; it's more common among those who had previously suffered pre-menstrual depression, which is associated with a similar (though much smaller) fall in hormone levels. Post-natal depression isn't just a consequence of hormone balance, however; the experience of the birth and feelings about looking after a new baby are also important. If your attitudes are positive, you might just feel tired; if they're negative, you're more likely to feel unhappy.

When hormone levels decline at menopause, many women become vulnerable to depression. When menopause is artificially rapid after hysterectomy when there is removal of the ovaries, depression is very common indeed; some degree of depression develops in over half the women in this situation, a frequency far greater than that after other types of surgical operation. But once again, an important factor in determining the way you feel is your attitude to the operation and to losing your ability to have children. Women who feel less feminine or less worthwhile as people because of their loss of fertility are more susceptible to depression after hysterectomy or menopause. After the period of rapid hormone change and adaptation is over, women achieve a new equilibrium, and depression and anxiety become less common.

Depression and other forms of mental or emotional turmoil are neither inevitable nor unavoidable at these times. A healthy lifestyle which sustains the underlying balance of the body will go a long way towards preventing distress. Good nutrition, which ensures that the micronutrients we need for optimum function are always available in sufficient quantities, is especially important. So don't go on a calore-reduced diet because you feel bad about yourself, or start eating junk because you can't be bothered to look after yourself; that way, you make everything worse.

Plan for the vulnerable times by looking after your needs before they become critical. Don't try to initiate a more active lifestyle at a point when your motivation is unpredictable; get into the habit of it earlier in the month. When you're pre-menstrual, tune in to the energy that's available to you and use it in physical activity so that your emotional stress levels stay low.

Bursts of energy are common during the pre-menstrual period. Many women report that they feel lethargic and get less done, but studies using objective measures like pedometers, which record the amount of walking, show that this is an illusion; we're actually more physically active. I've noticed that I tend to get irritated with chaos a couple of days before my period, and I'll dash round cleaning the house, sorting out the debris that accumulates over the weeks when I can ignore the mess. I used to think that I was particularly untidy when I got pre-menstrual but when I actually examined what was going on, I realized that I was just more aware of it. I enjoy isolating myself and getting to grips with practical tasks—preferably to a background of wild, passionate music—when I'm in that frenetic state of mind. Now I know about it, I plan my activities to fit.

Once the period starts, energy falls. A quiet day early in the period can feel marvellous. This is a time for relaxation. The menstrual hut in which women of some primitive cultures are relegated away from the men of the tribe during their period often seems to me a most appealing concept; I want to lie around, free from my everyday duties so that I can chat with other women when I'm having my period!

When you recognize and use your emotional and mental cycles to enhance your life, you can build a positive pattern. Trying to deny the relevance of your hormones to the way you feel is a route to frustration. Acknowledge the strong and valuable qualities of each part of the cycle to get the maximum benefit.

It's a mistake to focus on the unpleasant aspects of these fluctuations. If we anticipate distress, we're more likely to feel it; if we think the physiological changes in our bodies are going to cause problems, we'll be more likely to create them. While emphasis on pre-menstrual misery makes it greater, recognizing pre-menstrual sensitivity and energy allows us to make the best use of it. If you keep a diary which helps you to understand how your feelings and abilities change over the course of the month, you'll learn how to respond to these changes and plan your life accordingly.

Beliefs and expectations have a strong influence on our perceptions of what's happening in our bodies. If you are convinced that your reactions are uncontrollable, that's what you're likely to experience; if you see them constructively, as potentially useful, you'll feel better and function more effectively. Similarly, if you anticipate pain, you will suffer more.

This is especially important for women who are about to experience childbirth; you'll have a better time and experience less pain if you believe that any pain will be manageable than if you're afraid it'll be more than you can bear. It helps to go to classes where you're taught how to keep pain to minimum so that you know you have some control over it, to talk to women for whom childbirth has been a good experience, and to read books (such as some of Sheila Kitzinger's tremendous output) which describe coping with childbirth in a positive way. By doing this, you can teach yourself to experience less distress; if you do the opposite, and focus on pain, you're likely to suffer more.

Whatever your situation, always focus on what you want to

achieve and how you're going to achieve it. Look where you want to go, not at the potential problems you may encounter. Taking note of possible difficulties and responding appropriately is different from wallowing in distress: you can acknowledge the difficulty but pass on quickly to focus on your intentions. You may be functioning slowly if your hormones are in a balance that induces slowness, as in late pregnancy, but you're still functioning and still making progress. Don't waste your energy fretting about what you might have been doing if your hormone were in a different balance.

When your hormones are in tune with your aims and activities, you'll get the best from life. This is the reality of holding the conductor's baton: you're not totally in control of what the hormone orchestra is capable of producing but you're certainly in control of the harmony! Go with the music; don't fight it but recognize it and respond to it. Tune in to your body's powers to enjoy living to the full.

CHAPTER EIGHT

Living on a Roller-Coaster

Being a woman means living on a hormone roller-coaster. Life is not stable; our bodies and feelings change constantly. We don't have the same energy level, at all levels, every day, but the demands of our lives often do not take account of this. We may sometimes wish we could emulate the predictable performance and requirements of automata but we're not machines and it can be difficult to accommodate the limitations that hormone swings create.

In adolescence, our overall body state fluctuates wildly as our hormone cycles develop and stablize. Those who've brought up adolescent girls will be all too familiar with the crazy ups and downs, the childish dependence that suddenly changes to amazing adult insight. These emotional and behavioural swings are inevitable when the underlying equilibrium is so uncertain.

Come adulthood, the world expects constancy but as women we don't feel it and we can't reasonably expect to, unless our hormone fluctuations are dramatically suppressed by medical means. The mental changes described in the last chapter, coupled with the familiar physical changes, make us vary from week to week and from month to month. This is our nature and no matter how constant the demands on us, we have to come to terms with what we really are.

Parenthood brings yet another set of changes that although more culturally acceptable are often personally unacceptable: accommodating the fluctuations of pregnancy and the re-balancing period after having a baby requires that we be tolerant of ourselves. Then menopause demands adaptation to another phase of change until we reach the 'Indian summer' of post-menopausal stability.

Our changing abilities, strengths and weaknesses, needs and

desires, require that we understand ourselves and acknowledge our personal realities. But there is no need to be crippled by feminine nature. We are not in any way inferior because of it.

Serious imbalance can, however, be crippling. It can seem to start quite suddenly and apparently unpredictably, and we may seek recourse to medicine in our struggle to cope. Unfortunately, the consequences of such intervention are sometimes worse than we anticipate.

Stress, illness and drug therapy can make us particularly vulnerable to hormone disruption. Sudden, acute or rapidly worsening loss of hormone balance can often be related to specific causes that may demand special action.

Every woman who is susceptible to hormone problems knows they get worse with stress. When we're under stress, our bodies secrete a range of hormones which interact with our sex hormones and affect their metabolism. Usually we're able to acknowledge what's going on and it may be enough for us to take care of ourselves with plenty of rest, regular gentle activity and a healthy diet to ride out the high-stress period without damaging ourselves. But sometimes stress can precipitate illness and the whole system can run downhill frighteningly fast.

During menopause, we become extra-sensitive to stress effects. If we haven't taken sufficient care of ourselves during the years leading up to menopause, we may not have the reserves to cope and we become unable to weather the changes we experience. Some women become hypertensive, develop allergies and food sensitivities, or run into other common problems of aging in our culture, such as diabetes. Such symptoms may add to imbalance in themselves, or lead to the use of drugs which can create further imbalance.

Under these disrupting circumstances, a normally adequate diet may become inadequate. Your body may not be capable of maintaining its equilibrium and you may not get the nutrients you need or you may excrete more than you should. But to choose appropriate action to restore health, you need to understand the underlying problem.

One type of problem that is increasing rapidly in our polluted world is allergy. This can have devastating effects on hormone balance. Food sensitivity, in particular, will disrupt your balance by altering the body's ability to make use of the nutrients in the food you eat. Such sensitivity seems to increase as we get older, and may get worse very rapidly during adolescence and menopause. Periods of major hormone change make us more susceptible to the allergens in food and the environment; we may put our problems down to change of life but that could be just one aspect of it. If we can recognize and deal with the allergy, we will be able to cope with other aspects of the change more easily.

Food sensitivity and allergy are especially likely to develop when we're already short of some of the important nutrients that support our hormone balance. Essential fatty acids, in particular, help to protect us from hormone problems but we may fail to absorb these properly if our digestive systems aren't working properly. The deficiency that develops makes matters worse because EFAs help prevent allergic reactions. I've known many women who had the most dreadful PMT until they were able to find a diet that suited them and allowed their bodies to absorb the necesary micronutrients in sufficient quantities.

If you suffer from chronic diarrhoea, colitis or irritable bowel, the chances are you'll suffer from symptoms of hormone imbalance. And when your hormone problems are at their worst, your gut symptoms will be at their worst too. Food sensitivity is often at the root of such problems; Maryon Stewart and her co-workers at the Women's Nutritional Advisory Service find that about one in ten of clients with the worst PMT symptoms are sensitive to everyday foods, especially wheat. When they cut the offending foods out of their diet, their PMT improves tremendously.

But there is a danger here. It's all too easy to attribute too many symptoms to too many foods, and restrict your diet so much that you run into more deficiencies. If you suspect food sensitivity, always test foods carefully to see how you react to them; cut the most common culprits out of your diet completely and then, when your health improves, re-introduce them one at a time so that your diet remains as varied as possible.

Wheat products—bread, cakes, biscuits, breakfast cereals, pasta and anything made with wheat flour—are frequent causes of chronic gut problems. If you decide to eliminate these foods from your diet, you may find you feel much better and that your hormone balance improves quickly. You're also likely to gain weight if you're thin, or lose some of the excess if you're fat.

Elimination diets such as these are not simple. You need to identify every source of even the smallest amount of the substance you suspect could be causing your problems if you're to be sure of discovering whether you react badly to it. If you give up wheat, ensure that you get plenty of complex carbohydrate from other sources and eat other types of grain food to provide the nutrients you need. Step up your intake of rice, potatoes and buckwheat spaghetti to balance your diet and avoid hunger.

Milk and dairy products are also common allergens that are linked with hormone imbalance. For many people they're difficult to eliminate from the diet because they are found in so many prepared foods. Read labels carefully, looking for tell-tale words like casein (milk protein) and lactose (milk sugar). Try giving up milk and cheese and substituting soya products when necessary. You can get the nutrients these foods would normally provide from alternative sources: tinned fish or tiny fish like whitebait, where you eat bones and all, can contribute the calcium you need, while regular exposure to sunshine and regular exercise will help your body to absorb and use it.

The list of foods tht can precipitate allergic symptoms in sensitive people is almost infinite. If you suspect that your hormone problems could be related to food allergy, get a book on the subject—Peter Mansfield's *Chemical Children* (Century) is very good. Use it to design test diets that allow you to identify the cause of the problem. At the same time, step up your intake of essential fatty acids; use evening primrose oil supplements and aim to eat oily fish such as herring, pilchards, salmon, sardines or whitebait every day until your symptoms improve. Vegetarians and vegans should buy linseed (Linusit Gold) and incorporate it into nut dishes.

If you want more information on this aspect of the hormone question, contact the Women's Nutritional Advisory Service at PO Box 268, Hove, East Sussex BN3 1RW. Maryon Stewart's book *Beat PMT Through Diet* is based on the work of this valuable organization and includes much helpful detail; I strongly recommend that every woman with intractable PMT should study this book.

For some people, food sensitivity and problems with nutrient absorption can be dramatically improved by careful food combining. The Hay system, described in *Food Combining for Health* by Doris Grant and Jean Joice (Thorsons), helps many people with digestive problems and can be useful for a variety of chronic illnesses. Basically, this is a way of eating that separates different types of food, so that you eat protein foods at some meals, carbohydrate and grain foods at others. Some women feel very much better when they eat this way, and hormone problems diminish as the whole body improves.

Nutrient balance can go awry whenever the elimination of minerals is increased. In general, whenever the output of urine is increased, there's likely to be a risk of deficiency of magnesium and potassium, which are very important in maintaining a healthy cardiovascular system as well as a stable hormone balance. Some types of medication or illness can reduce their levels in the body.

Increased urine production is one symptom of diabetes. Although this may disappear when the condition is under control, the filtration systems of the kidneys are often damaged. Diabetics will tend to lose magnesium and other minerals in their urine and need to take compensatory action to prevent hormone problems and other forms of health disruption.

Dr Katherina Dalton has written that the only men who can really identify with PMT sufferers are diabetics, because they too suffer hormone changes which affect their mental state and all their body systems; I would go further and suggest that many diabetics are in a very similar state of hormone imbalance much of the time and treatment for PMT is appropriate for both male and female diabetics! For the woman, her problems are doubled; but she can largely overcome them by judicious use of food supplements.

Sugar Plus, made by Nature's Best, will help reduce PMT at the same time as reducing diabetic symptoms; but take care when you experiment with it and try to work with your doctor or diabetes clinic. Your insulin needs are likely to decrease when you take this food supplement and you may have to reduce the dose of your medication to allow for this. This is a beneficial step to take for your long term health but in the short term, you'll need to be careful about your blood sugar balance. If you're worried about taking a supplement with such direct effects on blood sugar, the least you should take is extra magnesium. Diabetics will also benefit from a diet that is high in pulses (peas and beans) and essential fatty acid supplements.

Most drugs which increase urine production (diuretics) will tend to increase excretion of potassium and magnesium, making you more vulnerable to hormone problems. You may have been told you have to take these drugs because you have high blood pressure and are at risk of heart or blood vessel disease. If you can reduce your blood pressure by non-drug means, through increased rest, meditation, regular exercise, and diet modification (reduce salt, increase raw fruit and vegetable intake, give up coffee), your need for diuretics should disappear and your long term health will be much better.

Drinking a lot of tea, coffee, or alcohol can cause deficiency problems related to excessive urine production. These everyday 'drugs' are all diuretics and tend to increase the elimination of magnesium and other minerals from the kidneys. Try to cut your intake to a minimum.

Steroid drugs, prescribed for allergic conditions and many other types of chronic illness, cause severe disruption of mineral balance within the body. Sex hormone systems are inevitably affected when this happens. If you can avoid using steroids completely, you will be doing yourself a favour. Contact Babs Diplock (a long-term sufferer and campaigner), 115 Chichester Road, Cleethorpes, South Humberside (0472 696722) or Steroid Aid Group, PO Box 220, London E17 3JR if you have to use these powerful and dangerous drugs. Always include a stamped addressed envelope and, if possible, a contribution towards finances, when you contact these people: they're voluntary organizations with very little money.

Oral contraceptives contain hormones which change your body's internal balance and increase your need for some nutrients. If you've been taking the pill or have had a contraceptive injection, you'll need extra vitamin B_6 to compensate.

Illness and stress increase your requirements for micro-nutrients, and deficiencies which make your hormone problems worse are often precipitated by the demands they make on your body. Fighting infections uses up a lot of vitamin C and zinc; if you're prone to infection, as well as PMT, try supplementing your diet with these nutrients and increasing your intake of fresh salads, raw fruit, and organic meat. Stress problems may be related to inadequate intake of B group vitamins; if this is true for you, you're likely to suffer hormone imbalance too. Make sure your diet contains plenty of foods containing B vitamins (whole grains are best) and take B group supplements if you think you're still running short.

Finally, pregnancy and breastfeeding increase your nutrient needs across the board. Women who try to deal with weight problems which develop during pregnancy by cutting back their food intake are especially vulnerable to deficits developing at this time. Don't ever count calories! Just change to a sensible diet in line with the recommendations in Chapters four and nine and eat well whenever you're hungry. As your body's internal nutrient balance improves and you regain your energy, you'll lose your excess weight.

Many women only become aware of hormone imbalance after taking synthetic hormones. Coming off the pill is often the trigger for the development of PMT, especially if you felt pre-menstrual for the whole month while you were taking it! The trouble with taking hormones is that they suppress the body's natural production and your own hormone systems may take a long time to recover from this artificial interference. If you're in this situation, you'll need to be particularly careful to take action to get your natural hormones into the right balance.

In view of the disruption that can be caused by taking hormone-based drugs, it's ironic that these are the treatments many doctors prescribe for hormone imbalance. Medicines prescribed for period pain, pre-menstrual symptoms, fibroids and menopausal symptoms may all contain substances closely related to natural hormones.

Severe period pain and heavy periods may be treated with variations of the oral contraceptive pill: Controvlar, Norlestrin, Ovran and Ovranette are favourite preparations. Women on the pill tend to have light periods with little pain because hormones in the pill prevent the normal monthly cycle. Many doctors believe, therefore, that it makes sense to prescribe these hormones to women who have difficult periods and who don't want to get pregnant. (Note: Controvlar cannot be relied upon to suppress fertility and should not be used as a contraceptive.)

This method of coping is usually effective to reduce symptoms but it exposes woman to all the potential problems associated with oral contraceptives. Serious adverse reactions include thromboses, stroke and other forms of cardiovascular disease. These reactions are rare but can affect women of any age. Occasionally they can be fatal. Other serious long term problems include increased risk of cancers, particularly breast cancer, developing many years later. These risks are greater the longer you take the pill, the higher the dose of hormones in it, and the younger you are when you start to take it.

In the shorter term, depression can be a very serious adverse reaction because it can lead to suicide. Surveys have shown that suicide is much more common among pill users than among women who use other forms of contraception. Pill users are also more likely to suffer from allergies, migraine, diabetes, liver problems and vaginal infections. Weight gain is another common side-effect.

If you want to know more about the risks of hormone-based contraceptives, read Dr Ellen Grant's book *The Bitter Pill* (Elm Tree Books). Dr Grant worked for the Family Planning Association and studied the pill from its earliest days of use in Britain. At first she thought it was the perfect contraceptive but as the years went on she saw so much suffering and so much illness among pill users that she became implacably opposed to its use.

My experience of the pill is that its effects build up insidiously. When I first took it as a student in the sixties, I was enthusiastic; it seemed so safe, so trouble-free. I didn't associate it with the gradual decline in my health. It was four years before I came to suspect a link between the pill and my symptoms of depression, obesity, migraine and recurrent vaginal thrush. No doctor had warned me about the risks, nor did anyone suggest I try to alleviate my symptoms by coming off the pill.

I hope that today, when awareness of drug side-effects is much greater, that nobody would go through the misery that I endured without coming off the pill. But my experience has taught me to beware of doctors who assure me that I won't have any problems with this or that brand, or that my symptoms are imaginary or nothing to do with the drug. Such assurances are usually based on wishful thinking combined with ignorance, not established fact. In reality, no effective drug is completely safe, and it's very difficult indeed to know for sure whether illness is related to the use of a particular drug—especially one that acts as a hormone, with widespread and subtle effects on body systems.

I must admit that some women say they feel marvellous on the pill, and few go as crazy as I did when they take it. But even those women who thrive on it may be damaged by it in the longer term. For some women, ovulation and periods fail to return after they stop the pill. The degree of natural hormone suppression that can result is unpredictable and its consequences uncertain. This can be distressing to those who give it up because they've decided they want to start a family. If you have taken the pill, always allow at least three months between stopping it and trying to start a family; use barrier methods of contraception (a cap or condom) in the meantime.

For other women, the natural cycle may return quickly but often with associated PMT. It's not unusual for women previously free from pre-menstrual problems to suddenly develop them when they come off the pill. The body has to find a new hormone balance as it recovers from the suppressant effects of the pill, and it may not be quite as good a balance as before.

If you ask your doctor for help with PMT, once again you could receive a prescription for hormones. The most commonly prescribed drug for PMT is Duphaston (dydrogesterone), a synthetic form of progesterone, or you may be given natural progesterone suppositories (Cyclosert). Side-effects of Duphaston include nausea, vomiting, breakthrough bleeding and weight gain; natural progesterone may also cause weight gain.

Clinical trials of hormone treatments for PMT suggest that it is effective for only 30 per cent of sufferers, and of no help at all for another 30 per cent. The remaining 40 per cent get partial symptom relief. This does not seem a rational form of therapy to me, because it does nothing to alter the cause of the problem; it merely creates an altered imbalance in the body. Nevertheless, progesterone is relatively innocuous and if it keeps your PMT in check, it's unlikely to do you any harm.

Many other gynaecological problems may be treated with synthetic hormones, and some doctors will offer them even when they have no idea what's wrong. They're the universal cure-all for 'female problems'. Doctors are encouraged in this belief by the authoritative doctors' reference book the *British National Formulary*, which says confidently: 'Progestogens are useful in many menstrual disorders. They are used in the pre-menstrual syndrome, severe dysmenorrhoea, and dysfunctional uterine bleeding to relieve pain and prevent or arrest bleeding ... Alternatively the combined oral contraceptives may be used.'

While these problems are likely to be linked with hormone imbalance, chucking in more hormones almost at random seems a crazy way to solve them. It's bad enough being on a hormone roller coaster, without making the hills higher and the slopes steeper. The consequences of such a strategy are uncertain and in the long term, they cannot be beneficial. If hormone therapy works at all, it will merely suppress symptoms; when you stop taking it you might well find yourself worse off than when you started.

Virtually every type of long term drug therapy causes health problems. This is because the body seeks to re-adjust itself to the balance that it had achieved before you started taking the medicine, effectively counter-balancing the effects of the drug.

When you stop, your body's counter-action continues, making your symptoms worse. However, if you take medicines indefinitely, the risk of side-effects increases. At the same time, whatever has been pushing your body's balance out of kilter and producing the symptoms that led you to seek medical help, is likely to continue to affect you. It makes much more sense to get to the root of the problem and treat it by natural means. The body's balance will return and symptoms fade if your needs are properly met.

When hormones are prescribed for short term problems, this sort of hazard does not arise. However, even short courses of potent hormones can be dangerous. One such situation is the use of hormones during pregnancy. Hormone imbalance in pregnancy can cause a miscarriage and for this reason, doctors have turned to hormone therapy in cases of threatened miscarriage. In some cases, the consequences have been tragic.

If anything presses home the warning that we should beware of interfering with hormone balance by chucking in synthetics, it is the DES story. DES (di-ethyl stilboestrol) is a synthetic form of oestrogen. Three decades ago it was the therapy of choice for women at risk of miscarriage, particularly in America, in the fashionable clinics of New England. Thousands of pregnant women were given DES injections in the belief that it would help them keep their babies.

All seemed well until these babies reached their teens. Then a series of previously-rare cancers were discovered.

As young women, some DES babies developed unusual reproductive system cancers. Many have had important parts of their reproductive systems surgically removed. Others are dead. Before long it was discovered that the boys whose mothers had been given DES had genital abnormalities too. Many are infertile. Subsequently it was found that the mothers also ran increased risk of cancer as a result of being given DES.

The vogue for DES to prevent miscarriage did not last long; although its dangers were not recognized for decades, it was quickly proved ineffective. But the trail of tragedy left by this hormone continued. Fed to chickens to make them grow faster, DES reached the diet of children in Puerto Rico, causing four-year-old girls to grow breasts and to menstruate, feminizing small boys. DES is still used as a growth promoter in cattle in some parts of the world and still turns up in beef products.

In Britain, DES was little used. But other potent hormone

products have been popular and have also caused damage far greater than their benefit. When American doctors injected oestrogens into pregnant women, British doctors gave synthetic forms of progesterone. These have been shown to cause deformities in babies. I have met women who, because they lost earlier babies, were treated with these hormones during later pregnancies. Imagine the distress they felt when the longed-for baby arrived at last—deformed. Sometimes surgery, often a series of major operations, can return the child to a semblance of normality, but the price for a treatment of such dubious efficacy is far too high.

Each of these types of hormone treatment is believed to be safe and effective by the doctors who use it. Time after time, they are proved to be dangerous. Sometimes it takes decades before the dangers emerge. The conclusion is clear: hormone treatments must always be assumed to be risky. For pregnant women, the risks are particularly serious.

Juggling with hormones by taking large doses of synthetic forms is a hazardous way of trying to re-balance your body. Reassurances are based on assumptions that may, in time, prove unjustified. In the sixties, when I took the pill, it was believed to be totally safe; now we know it's not, but many doctors prescribe it just as casually as they did twenty years ago. Other types of hormone treatment (such as hormones for threatened abortion and hormone pregnancy tests) are no longer used because they sometimes caused damage in the early foetus. But the belief that hormones can be safe and effective therapeutic medicine persists. It's a belief that history must make us question.

Apart from oral and injected contraceptives, the main use of hormones today is for menopause and bone loss after menopause. This is a controversial issue that I'll later discuss in detail in chapter ten.

Other drugs used for hormone problems include bromocriptine (Parlodel) and danazol (Danol). Bromocriptine stimulates the brain receptors for one type of transmitter, dopamine. This is the transmitter that's believed to be reduced when oestrogen levels are high. It may be prescribed for a wide variety of hormone-related problems, from PMT to suppression of lactation, for menstrual disorders and breast disease. Bromocriptine has many side-effects, including nausea, vomiting, constipation, headache, dizziness, drowsiness, confusion, hallucinations, dry mouth, leg cramps, and blood-vessel problems.

Danazol alters the levels of sex hormones by acting on the pituitary gland, and it's often used for endometriosis. Its side-effects include nausea, dizziness, rashes, backache, flushing, muscle spasm, hair loss, acne, and masculinization.

Bromocriptine and danazol change hormone levels by interfering with control systems in the brain. But their effects are not restricted to re-adjusting hormones because the pituitary and the dopaminergic transmission system don't just control sex hormones. Their overall impact is much wider and therefore potentially even more dangerous.

Finally, conventional medicine can offer a variety of drugs to alleviate symptoms without influencing hormone levels. These include the familiar pain-killers: aspirin, paracetamol, ibuprofen and the like, as well as diuretics, muscle relaxants, and tranquillizers. What you receive will depend on how your doctor interprets your description of your symptoms, and on his assumptions and prejudices. For example, if you complain of water retention before your period you might be given a diuretic and this will cause your kidneys to produce more urine. If you complain of nervous tension, you might be given a tranquillizer—especially if you happen to be weepy with PMT when you arrive in the surgery. And if your main problem is pain, you'll probably get a pain-killer.

None of these drugs solve the problem, although they may help you feel a bit better in the short term. And they all have disadvantages.

Simple pain-killing drugs like aspirin are usually quite safe for occasional use, although some people are allergic to aspirin as well as to ibuprofen. Paracetamol is less effective for period pain because it does not have the specific effects on prostaglandins that you'll get from aspirin or ibuprofen. Don't bother to consult your doctor for a prescription for pain-killers: he isn't likely to be able to give you anything more effective than these over-the-counter medicines. And don't bother to pay extra for a formulation designed 'especially for women' or anything like that—these are marketing tricks designed to get you to pay more for cheap drugs. Stick to straightforward ibuprofen or soluble aspirin B.P., taken with a large glass of water containing a small teaspoon of bicarbonate to reduce the potential damage to the stomach lining.

People with stomach or duodenal ulcers, or bleeding problems, should not take aspirin or ibuprofen. And pregnant women should also avoid them because they can cause problems for the baby. Asthmatics may react badly to these drugs too.

Diuretics, as I explained earlier in this chapter, could make your PMT worse by increasing the rate at which your body loses important minerals in the urine. You're likely to have no need of them if you follow the recommendations given in chapters four to six.

Muscle relaxants are sometimes used for period pain. These are related to travel sickness drugs, and are generally harmless for short term use. But they're only likely to help with spasmodic dysmenorrhoea—colicky pain in the lower abdomen.

Tranquillizers used to be the cure-all for women's problems. In recent years, doctors have become reluctant to prescribe them after finally acknowledging that they are addictive. They're OK for short term use (a couple of weeks), not more; but of course they won't help your hormone problems at all. They'll just stop you caring so much. If you do take tranquillizers for any reason, avoid driving or doing anything that requires careful judgement. Your brain will be fuzzed as though you'd been drinking and you're much more likely to have accidents. In some European countries, the penalties for driving after taking tranquillizers are as severe as those for drunken driving.

Other types of therapy are generally less risky than conventional medicine. Herbalism, acupuncture, homoeopathy and other alternative systems may well be capable of helping to re-balance your body. However, there's little objective evidence of the benefits of these approaches for hormone imbalance because alternative therapists don't receive the same financial support as doctors to do research. Conventional drug trials are financed by the drug companies out of their enormous profits; in fact, an increasing amount of all medical research is now funded by the drug companies. Naturally, the tests they fund are those that are likely to help sell their products.

The manufacturers of herbal remedies are at a tremendous disadvantage in relation to the multinational pharmaceutical companies. Herbs may well be helpful for hormone problems but their safety and effectiveness have not, to my knowledge, been thoroughly tested. One herbal remedy that you can get over the counter from some health shops is the herb *Agnus Castus*. It's popular in West Germany but little used in Britain. Agnus Castus is used for both pre-menstrual and period problems. Raspberry leaf tea is also said to be good for period pain and to help with birth. It's a pleasant drink, and to the best of my knowledge completely harmless, although it's best to take individual advice and to follow the instructions on the packet scrupulously. However, once again, there's a shortage of clinical evidence to support claims for the benefits of the traditional remedies such as raspberry leaf.

Many people believe that herbal remedies are inherently better than synthetic drugs. But we must not forget that herbs and plant extracts can be just as powerful and just as hazardous as modern drugs—indeed, many of the powerful drugs the doctor can prescribe are derived from old herbal remedies. Foxglove, used for centuries for heart problems, is prescribed today in a refined form for exactly the same types of disease as traditional healers used it for; it was a dangerous remedy then and it's still dangerous in the hands of conventional doctors. It can also be very valuable, and since there is no safe substitute, it can save life; but it can also kill. So if you use herbs, take care.

Herbs like *Agnus Castus* have one advantage over conventional remedies. They aren't likely to cause any long term disruption of your hormone systems. Whereas taking synthetic hormones may suppress natural hormone production, *Agnus Castus* is said to have the opposite effect, which is likely to make it safer in the long term. But taking any remedy, herbal or otherwise, is still a matter of dealing with symptoms rather than with causes, and it makes sense only as a temporary stop-gap while you wait for lifestyle changes to take effect.

In the long term, the best remedies are in your own hands. Treat your body in accordance with its design, and it will function properly, the way it is meant to. Balancing your hormones naturally will improve your overall health and personal effectiveness without unpleasant side-effects.

If you have been exposed to hormones, drugs, or an illness which leaves you in a state of severe imbalance, concentrate on the healthy state you wish to achieve, and do everything you can to encourage health. This means you should try not to focus on your symptoms; they will fade gradually, with the slow improvement in your overall state.

By all means use complementary medicine as part of your overall strategy. Competent holistic therapists will advise you on diet, activity, relaxation and other aspects of health care while doing what they can to help you recover from your immediate difficulties. There is unlikely to be significant conflict between my recommendations on natural hormone health and the advice that complementary therapists will give you. You might find that their support will help you in your efforts to achieve a healthier way of life.

Hormone problems that follow illness, stress, or drug treatment, can be solved with a balanced lifestyle. Progress may be frustratingly slow but you will see gradual improvement. Remember the essential features of a health-inducing lifestyle: a balanced, varied diet that provides high levels of nutrients; adequate regular exercise, daily if possible; sufficient rest and relaxation to allow your body to re-build depleted resources, and a way of life that provides emotional satisfaction.

It is crucial that you don't give up too quickly, before you can enjoy the results of your new focus on health. You cannot expect a rapid turn-around; your symptoms probably won't just go away as if by magic, especially if you've had problems for a long time. But what improvements you experience are likely to be maintained, and as you feel better you'll be able to do more and get more pleasure out of life.

Lifestyle changes designed to improve health are changes you should plan to make for the rest of your life. This demands that you make health a priority—something that really makes sense when ill-health interferes so drastically with everything you want to do.

In our culture, we pay lip-service to health care. We talk of health yet focus on illness; we concentrate on treating established problems rather than preventing them or changing the way we live so that the problems simply cease to exist. The only way we can hope to achieve long term health is by living in a way that creates health. Therapy is no substitute for the right lifestyle.

However carefully we arrange our lives, problems do arise. Unexpected pressures, trauma, and disease touch us all. But solving these problems doesn't demand a drastic change from the everyday care that we should take to safeguard our health; it just requires that we give ourselves more time and attention so that recovery is supported. When you're healthy and your body is in a good state of balance, you may be able to get away with carelessness about your diet or lifestyle for a short time. When you're not so well, you have to take more care. It's a simple and obvious truth that we ignore at our peril.

CHAPTER NINE
Fertility and Pregnancy

Tip-top health is your best guarantee of a trouble-free pregnancy and a healthy child. Pregnancy makes heavy demands on women and good nutrition is crucial both before conception and when the baby is growing. During pregnancy, hormone production rises to staggeringly high levels and the nutrients necessary for hormone health will be needed in greater quantities than at any other time in your life.

Medical progress and improved monitoring during pregnancy have reduced the risks of childbirth to a very low level, but the most effective action you can take is to reduce your personal risk by making sure all your needs and your baby's needs are adequately met. If you choose to have a baby, you have a responsibility to safeguard your health because this is what will determine your baby's health. Women who do not take sufficient care not only risk losing their babies, but increase the chances that their babies will be born disabled or that they will suffer from life-long illness.

The person with the most responsibility for your health is yourself; good health is the product of a properly balanced lifestyle. When your health affects another life as well as the rest of your family, you have to take it seriously. The factors that are important for a healthy pregnancy are basically the same as those that create hormone health when you're not pregnant.

A perfect pregnancy requires careful preparation. Once you have conceived, your body is on automatic pilot; your hormones, and your body state, are largely controlled by processes the baby sets in motion as it develops in your womb. The time when you have the chance to make the choices is earlier, in the year before you intend to conceive.

If your body is well-stocked with all the nutrients essential for good health before you become pregnant, your baby will have the best chance in life. Many of the child's body systems go through crucial stages of development during the very first weeks of pregnancy—weeks when you may not even realize you're pregnant or, if you do, you may often feel sick and unable to eat or take care of yourself as well as you normally would.

Those first weeks of pregnancy determine whether your baby is born perfect or not; whether your child is susceptible to infections or resistant to them; whether your pregnancy progresses to its proper conclusion with the result a thriving baby. All these factors depend very largely on the mother's nutritional status during early pregnancy. And this in turn depends crucially on her state before the pregnancy begins.

How old you are when you first conceive is less important than most doctors used to believe. What matters is that you should be as fit and well as possible. But if you are thinking about starting a second or later baby, you should first consider the spacing of your children. Archaeological evidence, and studies of primitive tribes like those from which we sprang, show that women in their natural environment tend to space their babies quite widely, usually conceiving only about once every four or five years. This gap between pregnancies allows your body plenty of time to recover from the physical demands of bearing children. In our society, where food is always plentiful, we can have babies closer together but statistics show that it's best to leave a two-year gap between them.

When you are considering pregnancy, you should anticipate your future needs. First, of course, you will want to be at your most fertile, to minimize the disappointment and distress that you'll feel if months pass without the longed-for signs of conception. While our natural cycles are designed to create the best conditions for motherhood, we are subject to the many stresses and assumptions of the modern world that interfere with this. These range from fashion, which dictates that women should be boyishly thin, to the work ethic, that insists that work comes first, often to the exclusion of the needs of women and their babies. Convenience technology and 'instant' food which tend to make many women excessively fat are also factors.

When our bodies are unable to cope with pregnancy, nature tends to protect us by making us infertile. Young girls do not become fertile until they have sufficient fat to nourish a baby throughout the nine months of its development in the womb and during breastfeeding after birth. Healthy women have at least 10 per cent more fat than men. This extra fat is laid down in adolescence; until the growing girl has sufficient fat, her periods will not begin and she will not be capable of conceiving. Similarly, starving women, who have lost their normal body fat, become infertile.

Unfortunately, nature's protective systems don't go as far as we might wish. There's a borderline state of inadequate nutrition which is sufficient to permit conception but not good enough to support the development of a healthy baby. Many women in Britain are in this borderline state and our disturbingly high proportion of handicapped children (one baby in fifty is malformed) reflects this situation. If the mother's nutritional state is not so bad that her baby is obviously malformed, it may still not be good enough for the development of a strong child with the best chance of surviving into healthy adulthood.

In our society, malnutrition often creates excessive fatness rather than thinness. The people with the poorest diets may get plenty of calories so that they can lay down fat, but most of these calories come from sugar and processed foods which have little nutritional value and are loaded with anti-nutrients.

Extremes of both fatness and thinness are associated with poor nutrition and hormone imbalance. So when you want to get pregnant, you should aim to be well-rounded, plump: neither fat nor thin. Forget the fashion model image of leggy boyish looks: boys can't have babies. Women should have curves. Of course, we are all made differently; if your build is slender, you may be light but perfectly healthy. The point is that women should not struggle to be skinny if they want to have healthy babies; it's very important to eat well in the months before you become pregnant. So if you feel you are either fatter or thinner than, ideally, you should be, make special efforts to eat the most nutritious food you can find in regular, well-thought-out meals and take daily exercise so that your body is able to make the best use of it.

We prepare ourselves for pregnancy in many ways, sometimes without consciously realizing what we're doing. Most women make sure they have a stable home and partner before considering pregnancy. Yet they may take it for granted that their bodies are in a fit state and neglect to ensure that the baby's most urgent needs—for the substances from which it creates itself— will be safely met.

If you are planning to have a baby, you should take care to

ensure that your own hormone systems are in the correct balance before you try to conceive. Our monthly cycles are designed to create a state of high-level fertility at regular intervals and if those cycles are not working as they should, fertility will fall. It is entirely predictable that widespread hormone problems will in their turn be associated with increased difficulty with conception. So if you have been suffering from PMT, irregular or heavy periods or any other signs of hormone imbalance, you should tackle these problems by the natural means described earlier in this book. When your hormones are in the right balance, you will ovulate regularly and the hormone-controlled preparation of your body for conception will work the way it is designed to do.

When you take action to get your hormones into the right balance, your weight will tend to right itself too. Fat women tend to produce too little progesterone in relation to their oestrogen, while thin women may produce too little oestrogen. Without sufficient progesterone, the changes in the second half of your menstrual cycle which create the right conditions for implantation of the fertilized egg may be threatened; without sufficient oestrogen, you will not ovulate regularly. But eating sufficient good organically grown wholefood to prevent you from feeling hungry, coupled with exercise to keep you fit, and as much rest as you feel you want, will get these systems working as they should.

Environmental pollution also creates problems for would-be parents. Not only can it interfere with proper hormone balance, as chapter five explains, but it can damage the germ cells produced by both prospective parents and harm the developing baby in the womb. Chemicals can affect women both before and during pregnancy; babies may be born with genetic defects or deformities depending on the nature of the chemicals involved and the time at which the woman encounters them. Men who are exposed to poisonous chemicals and toxic metals such as lead may suffer from infertility. The man's testes are very vulnerable to the effects of chemicals, which can cause a low sperm count or damage the sperm, altering genetic material or preventing them from swimming strongly enough to fertilize the egg.

It's impossible to avoid all toxic chemicals and environmental pollution, but you can improve your situation. Some of my suggestions for remedies may seem very drastic, but drastic action may be essential to protect your child's life and what can be more important than that?

First, think about the job you and your partner do and the area in which you live. Do either of you work with potentially dangerous chemicals, such things as solvents and pesticides? If so, change your job. Do you live in an area where the air is contaminated by industrial fumes or fumes from traffic on major roads? Move house. And since you are being put to so much trouble, add your voice to the demand for an environmental clean-up—it's our children who are going to suffer from an increasingly polluted world.

Then think about your home. Do you use chemicals, anything from paint strippers to fly killers? Stop using them. Don't have any woodwork treated against rot or worm. With a little thought you may be able to find natural ways of dealing with such household problems—dampness, for example, is often due to lack of adequate ventilation—and avoid chemicals altogether. Do you smoke? Give up—both of you.

I've discussed the pollution of food in chapter five; but you should also consider the pollutants in your water supply. Find out about your local water; contact Friends of the Earth if you don't know where to get the information. If you have lead pipes, change them; lead will damage your baby's nervous system. If you have a private water supply and copper pipes, check the acidity of the water with a kit from an aquarium shop; if the pH is below 7, replace your copper piping with plastic or get a treatment system fitted to make your water alkaline; otherwise you risk copper poisoning and your baby won't grow properly. Filter your drinking water through a reputable jug system if you have any reason to be dubious about it.

If you take any medicines for chronic illness, see if you can manage your health without them. There are natural remedies that will help you recover from most types of illness and the fewer drugs you take, the better for your baby. Cut your use of social drugs such as alcohol to a minimum.

By taking these actions, you will maximize your fertility and your chances of having a healthy baby. Your body state will be properly balanced and every organ and system will be working at its best so that when you are pregnant, the hormones that sustain the pregnancy will be produced in the right quantities.

Like the menstrual cycle and fertility, the whole process of pregnancy, birth and breastfeeding is controlled and co-ordinated by hormones. Follicle stimulating hormone (FSH) and oestrogen set the scene by causing an egg to ripen in the ovary. At around day 14 of the menstrual cycle, the ripe egg leaves the ovary to float down the fallopian tube. This is ovulation.

Hormone changes create an environment that increases the chances that the egg will be fertilized. They change your mood to make you feel sexy; they change your smell so that your partner finds you especially desirable. And within the neck of the womb, hormones stimulate the cells to create a special nourishing alkaline mucus which encourages sperm to swim through and meet the egg.

High oestrogen levels and this special mid-month mucus make sexual intercourse easy and enjoyable. With practice, you can judge when you are able to conceive by taking a little of this mucus on your fingers and looking at its consistency. When it's wet, slippery and almost clear, looking rather like raw egg white, your fertility is at its maximum. It's like this for a couple of days in mid-cycle, and if you want to get pregnant this is when you must have intercourse. Don't feel you need to go at it repeatedly; once a day is enough. More frequent ejaculation can reduce a man's sperm count so that he's less fertile.

Fertilization usually occurs within 24 hours of ovulation. After ovulation, the mucus becomes thicker, forming a plug at the neck of the womb which keeps sperm out. You're likely to feel less interested in sex as a result of this.

Right at the beginning of pregnancy, before any modern tests can demonstrate that you are pregnant, you may be aware of it. What you feel is the immediate reaction of your hormone systems to the implantation of the fertilized egg in the lining of the uterus; this leads to subtle changes in hormone balance that you may not be quite able to describe, but whose meaning you can interpret.

After about seven days, the fertilized egg attaches itself to the thick, spongy uterine wall. The egg itself secretes hormones; at this point the crucial one is human chorionic gonadotrophin, which prevents the corpus luteum, from which the egg sprang, from shrinking. This is important because initially it is the corpus luteum itself which secretes hormones, particularly progesterone. If conception has not taken place, the quantity of progesterone secreted by the diminishing corpus luteum declines rapidly until there is too little to sustain the uterine lining, and a new cycle begins with menstrual bleeding. When the egg is implanted on the other hand, it is essential this does not occur; so progesterone production has to continue to maintain pregnancy.

The ovaries and the tiny embryo thus co-operate to produce a balance of hormones that sustain the earliest stages of the baby's development. If your hormone levels aren't quite high enough, you may have breakthrough bleeding but still hang on to the pregnancy; if they're lower still, you lose the embryo with your menstrual blood.

During implantation, the fertilized egg puts out microscopic fingers into the endometrium, or lining of the uterus. These fingers grow into the placenta, which, as well as keeping the growing baby supplied with nutrients and removing its waste, produces large quantities of hormones. These hormones maintain the reproductive organs of the mother's body in the right state for each particular stage of her pregnancy and prepare them for future demands.

Early in pregnancy, the main hormone produced by the placenta is human chorionic gonadotrophin (HCG). This causes the ovaries to produce still more progesterone. Peak production of HCG is at about the 70th day of pregnancy, after which it falls to a constant value for the rest of the pregnancy. HCG is thought to be linked with morning sickness because there are high levels of this hormone in the bloodstream of women who suffer from nausea in early pregnancy.

It is at this point in the pregnancy that you may have problems getting enough nourishment to keep pace with the rate at which nutrients are being used to fuel the growth of the baby and the placenta, and the production of this massive hormone output. This won't matter at all if you were well prepared for pregnancy before conception. Eat dry toast, fruit and nuts, brown rice— whatever you can keep down. But avoid food with added sugar even if your appetite is low.

Later in pregnancy, the large and well developed placenta secretes the hormones that it previously stimulated the ovaries to produce. Oestrogens and progesterone are synthesised by the placenta from materials produced by the adrenal glands.

Oestrogens are important in all aspects of pregnancy, particularly for the health of the reproductive organs and breasts. High levels of oestrogen increase the thickness of the vaginal lining and cause it to secrete greater quantities of lubricant, which can increase sexual pleasure. Progesterone stimulates the growth of body tissue, including hair, muscles and also fat, an essential body store used for milk production. It raises the body temperature and metabolic rate and, late in pregnancy, it relaxes the joints and ligaments in preparation for childbirth. Progesterone alters the skin, sometimes making it oily and occasionally causing acne on the face and back which usually disappears spontaneously as the pregnancy progresses.

Acting together, oestrogens and progesterone stimulate the growth of the milk ducts in the breasts. Even during the first three months of pregnancy, the breasts begin to produce colostrum, the first milk; this may be secreted well before the baby is due.

Other hormones produced by the placenta include melanocyte stimulating hormone, which causes the skin to produce brown pigment (melanin) and turns the nipples brown. In some women, high levels of this hormone cause brown pigmentation on the face and thighs and a brown line running down the centre of the abdomen which usually fades shortly after delivery. You may find that you tan more easily when you're pregnant because of the action of this hormone. Human placental lactogen is another hormone, essential to milk production; its presence is used as a test of the efficiency of the placenta in late pregnancy. Relaxin, a hormone which is believed to be produced by the placenta, softens the cervix in preparation for the birth and relaxes the pelvic joints.

The hormone output during pregnancy is colossal, greater than anything you'll experience at any other time in your life. For example, the maximum production of progesterone when it reaches its peak during the second half of the menstrual cycle is still just a few milligrams a day; but towards the end of pregnancy it can climb to 250 mg a day. Progesterone output rises 50-fold or even more; oestrogens rise 20 to 30-fold. These dramatic changes inevitably affect the way you feel.

Most pregnant women are prone to wide swings of mood. Sometimes you'll feel depressed or panicky and you'll overreact to the slightest thing; but if your hormone balance is right you'll also experience a wonderful sense of calmness and contentment—the 'madonna' look—at other times. Progesterone is the hormone that's believed to produce this sense of calm; it relaxes you both mentally and physically.

As your body prepares for the birth itself, your hormone state goes through a new series of changes. One hormone in particular is crucial for the onset of labour: oxytocin. This is produced naturally by the pituitary gland in the brain. Prostaglandins, which are local hormones, are also involved in the birth and they stimulate the uterus to contract. Prostaglandins control pain and swelling at the cellular level.

Oxytocin is the main hormone that controls milk let-down, which is the emptying of milk into reservoirs near the nipple. Because of its dual role in stimulating uterine contractions and milk production, it helps the uterus to shrink back to its normal size after the birth and this happens during breast-feeding. When you breast-feed, therefore, your uterus returns to shape faster and your whole body recovers more quickly from the birth.

This massive output of hormones, coupled with the growth both of your baby and your own body, makes constant demands on your nutrient stores. For everything to work as it should, you need to be very well nourished from before conception until the end of breast-feeding. Hormone production requires a host of micro-nutrients and you must take care to ensure that you are not short of any of them. If the production of any of the hormones necessary for pregnancy, breast-feeding and birth is restricted by lack of nutrients, both you and your baby will suffer. Many of the complications of pregnancy are linked with inadequate hormone levels.

In earlier chapters of this book I've explained the necessity for adequate levels of nutrition for the maintenance of the normal menstrual cycle. Before you consider pregnancy, you should do everything in your power to get this right. You need to start off with the right hormone balance to create fertility and prepare your body for the demands to come.

During pregnancy, the same nutrients are needed in even larger amounts. If your body cannot produce sufficient progesterone, for example, you risk losing your baby. To guard against this, you must be sure you get all the nutrients that can protect against PMT, which is also linked with insufficient production of progesterone. To remind you briefly, the vitamins that are particularly important are the B group, especially B_6; vitamins C and E; the minerals magnesium, zinc and chromium, and essential fatty acids.

A good diet, as you know, is fundamental to health, and never more so than in pregnancy. When you may feel nauseous in early pregnancy you'll have to take special care to eat enough, because the demands on your body will already be high. Plenty of fresh organic vegetables, whole organic grains, organic wholemeal bread, nuts, and fresh and dried fruits are very valuable.

The growth of your baby and the placenta that sustains it will be taking yet another set of nutrients from your body. Calcium, iron, zinc and folic acid are especially important because these are needed in large quantities for the development of new tissue, the increase in your blood supply, and for the baby's bones. Iron and folic acid, with the vitamin C required to allow your body to absorb and use them, occur all together in green leafy vegetables.

If you're vegetarian, you may be told that you won't get enough iron, especially if your doctor believes that only the 'haem' iron in meat is properly absorbed. Don't be swayed: vegetarians are no more likely to become anaemic than meat-eaters because vegetable sources of iron contain more vitamin C which enhances iron absorption. Just make sure you get a wide range of vegetables, especially peas, beans and green vegetables, and that you always eat enough. Vegetarians who rely on cheese dishes or just take an ordinary diet without the meat, and strict vegans or rastafarians, can end up malnourished if they don't consider their diet carefully and make sure it's correctly balanced.

Eating a lot of animal products can be harmful during pregnancy. Heavy meat-eaters have higher levels of chemical pollutants in their bodies and more likely to become deficient in essential fatty acids. Meat dishes bought ready-prepared (chilled foods, pâté and cold meats) as well as certain soft cheeses are especially hazardous: they may contain high levels of bacteria such as *listeria* that can harm your baby. If in doubt, contact the Department of Health for an update. If you must have convenience food, choose vegetarian forms that don't contain animal products.

Replace animal products with vegetable foods such as nuts whenever you can, and if you eat animal-derived food, go for low-fat forms (toxins tend to cencentrate in fat), trim off all visible fat and remove the skin of chicken to reduce your chemical intake. Get your calcium from low-fat sources such as skimmed milk, low-fat yoghurt and fish such as sardines where you can eat the bones. Full-cream milk does provide calcium but the fat it contains is not helpful to you or your baby. Cold-pressed and unprocessed vegetable oils, and the fats in nuts and seeds, are much better because they provide the cis fatty acids that are essential for the production of prostaglandins and healthy cell membranes.

Fish is wonderful during pregnancy. It provides many

nutrients in a good balance. So step up your intake of fish—of any type except dyed fresh or smoked fish or irradiated shellfish. Irradiation destroys folic acid, which is important to your baby's development.

You should make a special effort to avoid all chemicals when you are pregnant. These can disrupt your baby's development and pollute your breast milk. Don't eat foods with added preservatives, flavouring and colourings; avoid canned and processed foods as much as possible and go for whole, fresh produce. Avoid white flour products or food containing sugar—it's more important now than ever that you eat organically grown wholefoods.

Mouldy food and anything that's a bit off, stale, or old should be avoided too. Some moulds produce poisons which can harm your baby. It isn't enough just to cut off the obviously mouldy parts; the fungi that make food musty or mouldy penetrate deeply and you can't be sure that you've cut them away. Throw food away if you're at all doubtful about it.

The increase in oestrogen and progesterone levels in your body can make you prone to some types of illness, especially diabetes and vaginal thrush. Guard against both these problems by refusing all sugar and other refined carbohydrates. Avoid refined carbohydrates such as white flour products, heavily processed breakfast cereals and sugar, which deplete your body of important nutrients, notably B-group vitamins and chromium, and make you more susceptible to diabetes and thrush.

Pre-eclamptic toxaemia (PET) is a potentially serious illness of late pregnancy that's due primarily to magnesium deficiency. Its first symptoms are excessive weight gain, water retention, and a rise in blood pressure. Magnesium is crucial for a healthy hormone balance, especially when the demands of pregnancy increase the body's need for this mineral. Magnesium deficiency makes women more vulnerable to stress, which can precipitate toxaemia. As chapter four explained, magnesium deficiency is widespread, a consequence of chemical farming which is made more severe by milling of wheat to produce white flour. Milling removes the bran and germ, both rich sources of magnesium.

I live on a farm and keep sheep and, as a shepherd, I am very conscious of the importance of magnesium. Ewes are highly susceptible to toxaemia when they're carrying twins, and the link with magnesium deficiency is well recognized. I guard against this by using magnesium-rich seaweed on my pasture; you can do the same by taking kelp tablets. I've often thought how odd it is that British doctors don't seem to know that toxaemia results from magnesium deficiency when sheep-keepers, vets and doctors in America regularly treat the condition with magnesium injections.

If you had problems with PMT before your pregnancy, you are probably chronically deficient in magnesium and you should make special efforts to ensure that you get more of this essential mineral. Eat plenty of organic wholemeal bread and take kelp supplements if you are in any doubt about your magnesium status.

If you regularly eat enough organic food and avoid anti-nutrients that affect your hormone status (see chapter five), your natural hormone levels should stay high enough to prevent problems in pregnancy. Many women, of course, fail to do this, and some doctors will try to correct the hormone imbalances that result with injections of hormones. These often do more harm than good.

Hormones are used to stimulate ovulation in infertile women, to treat threatened miscarriage, and to induce labour. Other uses of hormones have now been discontinued because of the damage they can cause; they used, for example, to be given for pregnancy testing until it was acknowledged that they could produce malformations in the growing foetus. Sometimes, women take hormones accidentally during pregnancy if they are on the pill and don't realize they are pregnant; this, too, can cause malformations.

The problem with hormones when used medically is that they constitute a blunderbuss approach which may be more than your body can handle. When ovulation failure is treated with hormones, many eggs may be released at once, causing a multiple pregnancy. Then, the reasons for the hormone imbalance that prevented ovulation in the first place can lead to difficulties in maintaining the pregnancy. It's much safer and makes more sense to correct any hormone imbalance by natural means so that ovulation takes place in the normal way, with (usually) just one egg released at a time.

Treating threatened miscarriage with hormones is becoming less common than it used to be because doctors now recognize that the risk of producing malformations in the baby is always present when hormones are given during pregnancy. Some synthetic hormones related to progesterone (progestogens) cause female babies to develop male sexual organs; others cause malformations of the heart, limbs and digestive system; synthetic oestrogens have caused cancer in the children of women who took them. The authoritative doctors' reference book, the *British National Formulary* comments: "Progestogens have been used in habitual abortion [a tendency to miscarry] but there is no evidence of benefit." It is tragic that these useless remedies have caused so much damage. In 1989, only one product was listed for habitual abortion: Gestanin, a progestogen.

Miscarriage is common; at least one in ten pregnancies end this way, to the great distress of many women. Probably one in three women miscarry during their first pregnancy. Usually it happens during the first three months and most of these pregnancies would never have developed properly because of abnormalities in the placenta or the foetus. The warning sign is bleeding; if you have both pain and bleeding, miscarriage is usually unavoidable.

When hormone imbalance is so common among women generally, it's not surprising that miscarriage is common too. Maintaining a pregnancy, as you will now realize, depends on the production of very high levels of many hormones. If your body has problems producing sufficient hormones for a healthy balance when you're not pregnant, the demands of pregnancy could easily be too great.

If you are at risk of miscarriage, drugs will not help. Instead, rest, eat well, and most importantly, DO NOT SMOKE! Smokers are twice as likely to lose their babies during pregnancy; their babies are less healthy at birth and more likely to die within their first year. Those who survive suffer more illness as children. Every mother wants her children to have the best start in life; that means *no smoking*.

Oxytocin (given as an intravenous drip) is the hormone that's most likely to be given to pregnant women whose labour is induced. Sometimes labour is induced using pessaries or gels containing prostaglandins.

Induction of labour with oxytocin used to be very common in the late 70s, until protests from women and exposure in the media caused doctors to desist. In some hospitals, induction was used to ensure that women had their babies at times convenient to the consultants—it was childbirth by the clock, between nine and five, weekdays only.

Because oxytocin is the natural hormone that causes labour to begin, it used to be assumed that artificial induction was quite safe. Unfortunately this is not true. The drip does not deliver hormones in the same delicate balance as the body's natural systems, so the body is not properly prepared for childbirth. Induced labour is often excessively violent and painful and women are much more likely to need epidural anaesthesia and forceps deliveries, which can be harmful to both mother and baby.

In some hospitals, women are induced if their babies are considered as little as a week overdue—even when they are perfectly healthy. When there is always uncertainty over dates, such readiness to induce seems foolhardy. If your baby doesn't arrive on time, you should not be surprised; 80 per cent are actually born after they're due and only 5 per cent come when they're expected. My mother swears I was born six weeks late!

There are times when careful use of oxytocin can be justified; for example, when labour is very extended and contractions have become too weak to finish the birth, or when the placenta is ceasing to function so that the baby is not getting the nourishment it needs. It can be given as a tablet that you put under your tongue and suck gently, or given directly into your bloodstream through a drip.

Very few deliveries actually need augmentation with oxytocin, so don't accept it unless you are totally convinced that your baby is seriously at risk without it. The drip, in particular, causes strong and painful contractions which may be bad for your baby as well as miserable for you. You're more likely to tear when your labour is induced, so you will almost certainly be subjected to episiotomy (a surgical incision between the vagina and anus) which will add to your discomfort after the birth.

It is possible to stimulate the body's production of oxytocin naturally, through sexual arousal. Extended sexual arousal and orgasm can raise the level of oxytocin in your bloodstream and may set off labour if you're due. Nipple stimulation is especially effective. During orgasm, the uterus contracts naturally, which is good for the muscles, but the contractions will stop again if your body is not ready for the birth. Intercourse will not harm the baby unless your waters have broken, when there may be a risk of introducing infection.

Once your baby is born, a new hormone balance develops very quickly. Without the prodigious production of hormones by the placenta, the levels of progesterone and oestrogen in your body fall. The rapid drop in sex hormones may be partly responsible for the depression that many women feel after their babies are born, but the whole situation—the demands of the new baby, broken nights, the sense of anti-climax when you're alone with the mucky nappies—may be quite enough to bring you down sometimes!

Hormones control the production of milk, just as they made your breasts capable of secreting it. Prolactin, a pituitary hormone, stimulates milk production; oxytocin makes the milk available to your baby. Even thinking about feeding your baby can be enough to make your breasts produce milk—another example of the close links between mind and body that we find throughout the whole endocrine system.

Just as thought can cause a surge of hormones, so emotional tension can interfere with hormone production; mental stress can lead to difficulties with breast-feeding. The right balance of hormones is once again dependent on the overall balance of your life. It's important, of course, to eat well and to avoid chemicals, because you want your baby to get the best possible nourishment; but it's also important to look after yourself in other ways, to rest when you feel tired, and to relax whenever you can. Your personal well-being has to have a high priority; your baby's health depends on it. Never mind if the house is a tip: let others sort it out, or ignore it; you have a new baby to care for and that means caring for yourself.

Because milk production is controlled by hormones, taking extra hormones will inevitably affect it. Some doctors prescribe the contraceptive pill or long-acting injected contraceptives to new mothers. If you accept these hormonal methods of contraception, your milk supply is likely to fail. And over the period when you can continue to breast-feed, your milk will be contaminated by sex hormones, with unpredictable effects on your baby.

When you're breast-feeding regularly, you are not likely to be fertile because your hormone balance will not be appropriate to supporting another pregnancy. This is nature's way of ensuring that you don't have too many babies in quick succession. Unfortunately it isn't 100 per cent effective and fertility sometimes returns faster than expected, especially if your baby isn't relying totally on your breast milk. To be safe, you should start using barrier methods of contraception when you resume intercourse after you're recovered from the birth.

In this chapter, I've been concentrating on the question of

hormones in pregnancy; there's a lot of information that parents-to-be should have that is not given here because hormone balance is only part of the picture. The whole issue of health before conception and during pregnancy has been studied in depth by the charity Foresight, the Association for the Promotion of Pre-Conceptual Care. Foresight have produced a range of booklets for would-be parents. These contain a wealth of detailed information designed to help those who have difficulty conceiving or who want to give their babies the best possible start in life. Contact Foresight by writing to the Secretary at The Old Vicarage, Church Lane, Whitley, Surrey GU8 5PN.

CHAPTER TEN
Menopause: Coping with Change

Menopause is the time when our periods cease. Often defined as the first complete year without periods, menopause occurs, on average, when women are fifty-two. For some women, the menopause can begin as early as forty; doctors call it 'premature' if it begins before the age of forty.

During the menopause, the hormone balance shifts from one which supports fertility to a stable pattern of infertility. Menopause, or as it is often called, 'the change' can be a time of total upheaval or you may sail through it, scarcely noticing the changes going on in your body. How you feel is a product of many interacting facts, not just the physical issues like the quantities of hormones in your body, but all the cultural, social and psychological implications of aging.

The menopause is more than the cessation of a body function that most women are happy to lose by that age. It marks the passage from youth to age and the feelings we have about it are closely tied up with our attitudes to growing older, to fertility and infertility, to beauty and wisdom. These are problem areas where people in many Western cultures flounder, trying to live by values that deny or distort biological reality.

Many women fear menopause as a miserable, difficult period from which they seem to anticipate emerging as bent and wrinkled old women, at risk of broken bones and deformity. Certainly this is the impression the medical literature gives, with its emphasis on oestrogen deficiency and osteoporosis. Nature, we are led to think, made a horrible mistake with women; we live far too long and our bodies weren't designed to cope. The influential American gynaecologist Vicki Hufnagel believes that the decline in oestrogen that follows the onset of menopause "is a deficiency state unique to humans because of our extraordinary longevity".

For those who see menopause in such a negative and pathetic light, it is inevitable that the response would be to interfere with nature by putting back 'deficient' hormones. What the natural design omits, human genius and technology can put back. Such beliefs imply that seeking to understand the situation in order to deal with problems by natural means is a waste of time and energy.

But menopause problems—when they occur—reflect the problems facing women in our culture. Suppressing them (as far as it's possible to do so) by replacing declining hormones can only be a partial, unsatisfactory solution. A holistic approach offers wide-ranging benefits and the opportunity to exert control for ourselves.

Far from being nature's mistake, I believe that menopause is one of her triumphs. The most incredible feature of the human animal is our brain: convoluted, sophisticated, capable of storing and manipulating massive amounts of information. As we go through life, we are (or should be) learning all the time, so that the oldest individuals in human groups accumulate valuable stores of experience, knowledge and wisdom. The survivors in primitive societies will tend to be those who are both lucky and perceptive; the contribution they can make is particularly great.

As our bodies age, child-bearing becomes increasingly onerous. There comes a point where the older woman can make more contribution to the ultimate survival of the group through her wisdom rather than her babies, so nature protects her from the risk of repeated pregnancy by changing her hormone levels to render her infertile. Because of the menopause, women have many more valuable years, an Indian summer of stability and uncluttered energy.

This transition is not always easy. After forty years in which reproductive imperatives may have been tremendously important in our personal lives, the cyclical fluctuations of our bodies and in our social lives, shedding the old pattern can cause stress. And if those forty years may have also involved neglecting and abusing our bodies and our health needs, we'll also be feeling the effects of the damage that causes. Menopause can also be the time when our past catches up with us and the future looks grim; a time of foreboding and loss.

Ours is a youth culture, for women particularly; whereas men look rugged when they carry the marks of experience, women whose faces lose the smoothness of youth are seen as just ugly. The eloquent lines of age, the outward signs of accumulated wisdom, are not appreciated; knowledge has replaced wisdom, technology superseded understanding. Our culture's stock of information is maintained on paper and disk, not in our heads. To see too far is to deny immediate profit. When wisdom falls victim to techno-culture, age has no value.

So, many women try to deny their age and reject the reality of change for as long as possible as they peer down the crumbling tunnel of their own decay. Inevitably, with every undeniable sign of transition, the psychological pain and fear increases. We sacrifice our faculties on the altar of assumption. The emotional charge is entirely negative, totally damaging.

No wonder women dread the menopause!

When attitudes such as these exist, depression is bound to be common. The link with attitudes has been supported by research which shows that women in very child-centred cultures have the worst time of it when they can no longer have babies. In America, Jewish women suffer the highest incidence of menopausal depression, other white women an intermediate rate, and black women the least. Anthropologists report that in pre-revolutionary China, where old women enjoyed a highly valued status, menopausal depression didn't seem to exist at all. According to anthropologist Clara Thompson, writing in *On Women* (New American Library, 1971), "By far the greatest hazards of menopause are psychogenical or culturally induced... A psychiatrist working in China reported to me that she had never seen a menopausal psychosis in a Chinese woman. This she attributed to the fact that in China the older women has a secure and coveted position."[1]

Cultural expectations play a large part in determining our experience of physiological change and the way we feel about any symptoms. This is much more important than is commonly realized. In our materialistic world we often ignore the psychological component of menopausal distress—even though it's on this level that it causes problems! Symptoms are only unpleasant if we perceive them as such; and if we react with fear, menopausal symptoms become more intense and more frequent.

Of course, the physiological changes that set all this off should not be dismissed. They do represent a far-reaching upheaval.

[1] Clara Thompson, *On Women* (New American Library, 1971).

Female sex hormones affect every cell of our bodies, and every reaction; their fluctuations can make us crazy or serene, energetic or despondent, strong or flaccid. And menopause is certainly a time of hormonal upheaval.

The number of egg cells in the ovaries declines steadily as we age until, at menopause, ovulation fails to take place. Follicle stimulating hormone rises to ten or twenty times greater than menstrual levels, trying to push the ovaries into their long-accustomed function. Progesterone, normally produced after ovulation, falls to an undetectable level. Oestrogen levels fall erratically and the proportions of the different hormone types change.

Luteinizing hormone, which is also produced by the ovaries, rises. Sudden release of this hormone is linked with menopausal hot flushes. Other hormones also fluctuate with these flushes, corticosteroids and other adrenal hormones in particular. Testosterone continues to be produced at a steady rate by the ovaries, apparently unaffected by the rest of the hormonal turmoil.

Although it seems that these changes are set off by the transition of the ovaries from egg-bearing organs to hormone-secreting glands, the ovaries are not the only determinants of the physiological pattern. Androstenedione, produced by the adrenal glands, is converted into oestrogen in fat cells. How much is available to the body to cushion the course of menopause depends on how much the adrenals can produce, how fast the body transports it or breaks it down, and how many filled fat cells there are for the final conversion.

Women who have had problems with hormone imbalance throughout their fertile years may look forward to menopause, expecting these difficulties to come to an end. But these women find they have the most difficult transition, their previous problems magnified, if they fail to act positively to change matters. Menstrual problems are strong predictors of menopausal symptoms. But just as it's possible to free oneself of menstrual problems, so appropriate action to balance the same hormone systems will help with menopause.

So what are these symptoms of menopause? For about one woman in ten, there are none apart from the cessation of menstruation. And despite the apprehension that many women feel in the years before menopause, 'change of life' produces very little change for the vast majority. Nevertheless, three out of four women experience hot flushes which are likely to occur over a period of two or three years.

Hot flushes are unpredictable in their frequency and intensity but they aren't in the least painful. They feel like a wave of heat spreading through the body, sometimes starting with tingling and accompanied by rapidly-spreading redness and sweating. They may be extreme, turning you beet-red, or quite mild, so that you just feel as though the room had become temporarily too hot. After the flush, which might last a few seconds or up to a couple of minutes, some women feel chilled because the body temperature can fall slightly.

Flushes can happen at any age and most of us are familiar with them long before we reach menopause. You've probably reacted to hot, spicy or meat meals by flushing; or to alcohol, infection, sudden excitement or embarrassment. The difference is that the menopausal hot flush, although shorter-lived than the others, can come on when you're just sitting quietly.

Hot flushes can be very bothersome if they happen frequently at night. Some women wake so many times during the night that they suffer from insomnia. In the daytime, the main problem is likely to be embarrassment; turning beetroot at a formal meeting, having to throw your clothes off, can be very awkward! But for most women, choosing layered garments that permit control of your temperature relatively easily will be enough to help you to cope.

Nervousness, temper tantrums, irritability, excitability and depression are all fairly common menopausal symptoms. Some women complain of dizziness and faintness, headaches and insomnia. Of course, these are all problems that are not uncommon at other times in one's life and it can be difficult to tell whether they're definitely related to the hormonal upheaval.

Weight gain, bloating and vaginal itching are the next most common problems of the menopause. The vagina, along with the breasts and other sexual characteristics, are oestrogen-dependent and as the level of this hormone falls, the tissues shrink. Vaginal dryness and soreness can make intercourse difficult. Less common symptoms include sore gums, joint pain, backache, muscle pain, hair loss or gain, dry mouth, and problems with swallowing.

It's obvious that many body systems can be affected by menopause, but also that those of us who see menopause as a source of great problems could attribute just about any form of discomfort to it. Some doctors react to almost any complaint from women between forty and sixty with, 'It's your age, the change of life.' You can believe this if you want to; with a holistic approach, you deal with the problem differently, whether it's down to menopause or not, because you focus on building up your health.

For some women, menopause is associated with loss of sexual interest and a marked decline in sexual activity. Between the ages of 50 and 60, about 40 per cent of women lose interest in sex. Yet research into this issue reveals that this need not be true; such sexual atrophy results primarily from attitudes and assumptions rather than from physiological change.

The purpose of sexual activity after menopause is pure pleasure: sex maintains and sustains happiness and closeness between people. So unless it is wholeheartedly desired *for its own sake*, the biological systems will cease to support it. Those who associate sex with babies are most likely to give it up when they are no longer fertile. When sex has seemed pretty boring anyway, menopause can be a good excuse for opting out of an unpleasant chore. Our culture denigrates sex for all except the young and those who internalize this attitude will readily reject their own sexuality when signs of age appear.

When sex is an important part of a loving relationship, menopause doesn't seem to affect it; in fact, for many women, it gets better than ever. Far from declining, sexual interest can increase after the menopause; freedom from the risk of pregnancy may allow the rebirth of pleasure and spontaneity. In many primitive societies, older women are considered particularly good sexual partners for young men because they're not sexually inhibited and their experience makes them good teachers.

Research into the question of sex and the menopause has shown clearly that continued sexual interest and activity depends on the way we feel and think about it. Women who have active sex lives retain their sexual interest. In some studies, the only significant predictor of a woman's sexual interest and activity was the presence of an interested partner.

The physiological changes, then, seem to be determined by psychological factors. And indeed, the timing of the changes reflects this. The majority of women have no oestrogen-linked vaginal symptoms for five years after the menopause—but many effectively give up sex when their periods cease. It seems that younger, fertile women can often put up with sexual intercourse without much suffering even if they're not interested in it; but older women must actually want it. If a woman doesn't want sex after the menopause, her vagina effectively becomes incapable of accepting coitus: thin-walled, unlubricated, no longer elastic, delicate and susceptible to infection. Intercourse then causes pain and problems.

The most serious of the long term problems that can afflict post-menopausal women is osteoporosis, or weakening of the bones. Bone loss begins immediately after the menopause. By the age of 70, 40 per cent of women fracture their wrist, hip or spine. Hip fractures, 80 per cent of which are associated with osteoporosis, are getting more and more common. Their consequences can be very serious, with 17 per cent leading to death within three months.

Compression fractures of the spine are another common effect of osteoporosis. The vertebrae in the old woman's bent neck and back may break and fuse, restricting her mobility and causing pain. A quarter of white women over the age of 60 in the US have spinal compression fractures.

Bone loss is linked with reductions in oestrogen and progesterone. If women are given either of these hormones, the rate of loss will slow down. But, as we shall explain, hormones are not the only important influences on the development of osteoporosis.

Natural ways of coping with the menopause can prevent the development of long term problems including osteoporosis. Predictably, all aspects of our lives are involved in this problem, and the increase in serious symptoms reflects the multitude of changes that shape the way we live. Around menopause, living in a way that isn't right for our bodies can have particularly nasty consequences so it's crucial that women should take care of their health needs at this time.

Eating well, of course, is vitally important. Without sufficient good food, none of our body systems function as they should. If we don't get the minerals and vitamins we need to create hormones we can expect them to decline more precipitously than they need do. And if we don't feed ourselves the constituents of strong and healthy bones, they will eventually weaken.

The right diet for menopausal women isn't fundamentally different from that for younger women, but some aspects of diet deserve special emphasis. A diet of organic wholefoods will prevent the constipation and weight gain that bothers some menopausal women and will help protect you from the food sensitivities and other allergies that often flare up during this hormone hiatus. Apart from this, the foods that you need are those containing the minerals boron, magnesium, zinc and calcium, which are all crucial for healthy bones.

Boron has recently been shown to be essential to older women. A study of women aged 48 to 82 living in a metabolic unit run by the Human Nutrition Research Centre in North Dakota, showed that extra boron (3 mg per day) reduced excretion of calcium, phosphorus and magnesium, thus protecting both the bones and the cardiovascular system. Boron increased body levels of both oestrogen and testosterone, which together maintain sex drive and potential as well as preventing menopausal symptoms. Within eight days of boron supplementation, mineral and oestrogen metabolism improve dramatically. Arthritis and rheumatism are also reduced with a high boron diet.

Boron is found in foods of plant origin, especially fresh fruit and vegetables. Vegetables contain 13 micrograms per gram of boron, dairy products 1.1 micrograms, cereals 0.92, meat just 0.16. So the best way to raise your boron intake is to eat more vegetables. Make sure they're fresh, preferably raw; if you can get organic vegetables, go for them because they contain higher levels of minerals.

Dairy products and fish bones contain high levels of calcium, but many women with osteoporosis cannot tolerate some dairy products because of sensitivity to lactose. Low-fat yoghurt is a much better source of calcium than whole milk or cheese because the lactase is pre-digested by the lactobacillus it contains. So if you can incorporate a large helping of natural yoghurt in your daily diet—ideally eaten with fresh fruit such as banana, pears, apricots or peaches—you'll be doing yourself a great favour. Whole fish such as sardines, whitebait, pilchards (where you eat the bones) and tinned salmon are very good too, also brazil nuts and almonds, beans, peas, and watercress.

High magnesium foods are described in chapter four, but to remind you, here's a shortlist: eat whole grains, beans, peas, nuts, seeds and green vegetables. Conveniently, these are the foods that also deliver the other nutrients you need.

Zinc, too, is found in nuts, organic whole grains, egg yolk, peas and beans, but the richest sources of all are oysters and red meat.

Vegetarians are susceptible to zinc deficiency unless they make sure they eat plenty of vegetable proteins.

Foods to avoid are bran, rhubarb, beetroots and spinach. All these can reduce mineral absorption. Tea, coffee and alcohol will also reduce the amount of minerals, particularly zinc, that you get from your food. Avoid drinking more than one cup or glass of each per day, and never drink tea with your meals.

Osteoporosis has been linked with a diet high in meat and dairy foods. This sort of diet—very popular in western industrialized countries where osteoporosis is most common—is often high in convenience and processed foods which deliver a lot of anti-nutrients and worthless calories. It's also associated with cancer, especially breast cancer, which afflicts one woman in nine.

Changing your diet to protect your bones cannot be done too early. Although osteoporosis causes serious damage after the menopause, building strong bones in the years before the change will protect you in later life.

Other menopausal symptoms can be reduced with the right diet. Vitamin B_6 and vitamin E are beneficial; try supplements (50–100 mg per day of vitamin B_6; 50–500 units of vitamin E) if you're bothered with hot flushes. Experiment with the dose to find how much suits you. Vegetable oils, nuts and seeds, eggs and green vegetables contain vitamin E.

Many women are worried about their weight in the middle age. The bad dietary and activity habits of earlier years catch up with us then, when metabolic rate tends to slow down and the spare tyres accumulate around the midriff. But the evidence on weight is reassuring: it's a good idea to stay quite plump and not to struggle to achieve the skinny looks of a young girl. Menopausal symptoms are less severe in plump women and osteoporosis less common because oestrogen levels stay substantially higher. The most badly afflicted women are those who are thin: prepare for menopause by making sure you're not thin! If you are prone to thinness, always eat plenty of good food, avoid getting stressed, get plenty of rest and meditation, give up smoking, and build up your body with activity.

Making sure you build healthy bones and muscles, however, it not the same as putting on weight. Excess body fat predisposes us to many chronic illnesses including heart disease, high blood pressure, diabetes and cancer. If you do have a real weight problem then you should look to your diet. But don't count calories! Just give up unhealthy foods like sugar (you don't need any sugar), biscuits, cakes, pastries, pies and puddings, and cut back on all animal and processed fats. Chips are out if you want to stay glamorous and healthy well into old age!

The most important lifestyle change for reducing excess fat is to take more exercise. This, too, protects you from osteoporosis by strengthening the bones. Take a long walk every day and if possible, take other forms of exercise too. In Denmark and Holland, where women of all ages rely on their bicycles for transport, fat people are rare. Forget the car—get on your bike!

The more exercise you take, the better, so long as you don't strain your muscles and joints. As we age, recovery takes longer and it doesn't make sense to go in for exercise binges that make you sore for days. Go at it gently but steadily; even half an hour's walking three days a week will provide substantial protection, cutting bone loss to negligible levels.

Exercise can be very helpful if you suffer from hot flushes or cold hands and feet. To train your body for better temperature control, or to adapt more easily to changes in internal temperature, start an exercise regime that's sufficiently demanding to make you feel hot and keep you sweating for 10 minutes or more. Any kind of exercise will do so long as it makes you sweat: walking uphill, aerobics, weight training, dance, fast cycling, running, or even jobs around the home like sawing wood or cleaning the windows. This sort of excercise will help keep you strong and young; it will make your hair shine and your skin glow. When you get your circulation going with hard exercise, you'll experience many benefits. But do be sure not to over-do it; always do about half of what you think you're capable of until you are sure of your capacity for demanding activity.

Try not to pollute your body with cigarette smoke and other poisons; this is always dangerous, but particularly so for middle-aged and older women. Smoking is definitely linked with osteoporosis as well as cancer and heart disease. Don't do it! Make up your mind to give up; get help from a hypnotherapist or anti-smoking group if necessary and help yourself during the withdrawal period by refusing coffee (which enhances the misery of nicotine withdrawal) and taking plenty of outdoor exercise.

Aluminium is another pollutant that grows in importance as we age. It damages the brain causing dementia and it interferes with mineral metabolism, causing bone damage. Replace your aluminium cookware with steel and don't take antacids that contain aluminium (brands include Alu-Cap, Aludrox, Actonorm, Andursil, Antasil, Asilone, Dijex, Diovol, Gastrils, Gastrocote, Gaviscon, Gelusil, Maalox, Mucogel, Polyalk, Polycrol, Prodexin, Siloxyl, Sylopal, Synergel, Topal, and Unigest). Aluminium is added to the water supply in many parts of the country. Ask your local water company whether yours is polluted with aluminium; if it is, filter your drinking and cooking water through a jug or ion-exchange system.

Vaginal problems that develop with menopause are linked primarily with feelings about sex, as I explained earlier. But there are some measures you can take to minimize vaginal soreness and itching. The first is to avoid soap, bath preparations and detergents which may harm the delicate membranes. I discovered that I suffered from dreadful itching and discharge when I washed my underwear with detergents that contained enzymes and other chemicals. Changing to Ecover washing powder cured the problem. Sensitivity to the constituents of washing powder is very common among women; we're doing a favour both to ourselves and to the environment by avoiding damaging detergents. Second, don't use any soap, cleanser or disinfectant around the sex organs, and don't add bubble paths or perfumes to your bath water. Wash gently with warm water, adding a little salt and distilled vinegar to the washing water if you wish.

Vaginal dryness is best countered with plenty of pre-coital sex play. Don't have a bath too soon beforehand: even if you don't use soap, a bath will tend to dry the membranes. Mental preparation with a sexy story helps; the best physical preparation, in my view, is a slow massage. But most important is desire; lubrication doesn't happen easily without it.

Lack of lubrication is often a mental, rather than a physical problem. If you're losing interest in sex, this may reflect difficulties in your relationship. Anxiety, anger, resentment and distrust are the most powerful anti-erotic forces. If your sex-life is going sour, you might benefit from talking through your problems with a counsellor; contact your local branch of Relate for sympathetic help.

Of course, it may be that all you need to solve your problems is a tube of lubricating jelly, such as KY. Keep it by your bedside: it's good stuff!

The option your doctor may offer you if you look for medical help with menopausal problems is hormone replacement therapy (HRT). This usually means a regime of oestrogens and progestogens (synthetic substances related to progesterone) which you take on a cyclical basis like oral contraceptives. The progestogen content will cause your uterus to shed its lining on a regular basis, as though you were still having periods.

In its early days, HRT meant oestrogen therapy alone, because it's the oestrogens that help with menopausal symptoms. Then, in the mid-seventies, it was discovered that oestrogens on their own could cause cancer of the endometrium, or lining of the womb. Progestogens are added to prevent this problem but not all of the combined preparations contain sufficient to fully oppose the effects of oestrogens. Women who have had hysterectomies can take unopposed oestrogens; they are better off without progestogens, which tend to reduce the benefits of HRT and may make menopausal symptoms worse for a while. There is a possibility that combined preparations may increase the risk of cardiovascular problems but they have not been prescribed long enough for anyone to be sure.

Both synthetic and natural oestrogens are used. Natural forms are preferable because they are less likely to lead to high blood pressure or thrombosis. These hormones are usually prescribed in the form of tablets, though injections and transdermal patches, through which hormones penetrate the skin, can also be used. Oestrogen creams are also used for vaginal problems. Brand names are given in Table 3, on the next page.

HRT can help with hot flushes, bone, joint and muscle pains, and can improve mood. The oestrogen component improves vaginal dryness and may increase sexual interest, but women on HRT do not respond with more frequent sexual activity or more orgasms. HRT prevents osteoporosis only while you continue to take it; it offers no long-term protection against broken bones.

There has been a lot of publicity about HRT that suggests that it can keep you young forever, preventing hair loss, wrinkles and all the other changes of aging. Actress Kate O'Mara is one advocate who's particularly fond of making public statements to this effect. But there's no evidence to support such benefits; HRT is not the elixir of youth. It doesn't prevent wrinkles or dry skin.

One curious facet of drug therapy for menopausal symptoms is the very large placebo effect. About a third of women will experience substantial improvements when they take placebos, or dummy pills. Just believing in the treatment has a dramatic effect. What this implies is that your mental attitude and your beliefs make a very large contribution to your symptoms, and to recovery from them. So when your friend enthuses about how well she feels on HRT, just remember that it may not be the

Table 3

Preparations used for hormone replacement therapy

Brand Name	Hormone Content	Comments
Prempak-C (tablets)	natural oestrogen plus progestogen	probably safest preparation for women with intact uterus
Estrapak 50 (tablets)	synethetic oestrogen plus progestogen	for women with intact uterus
Menophase (tablets)	synthetic oestrogen plus progestogen	"
Trisequens (tablets)	synthetic oestrogen plus progestogen	progestogen content may not be sufficient
Cyclo-Progynova (tablets)	natural oestrogen plus progestogen	inadequate progestogen content
Hormonin (tablets)	natural oestrogen	for women who have had hysterectomy
Progynova (tablets)	natural oestrogen	"
Ovestin (tablets)	natural oestrogen	"
Premarin (tablets)	natural oestrogen	"
Benztrone (injection)	synthetic oestrogen	"
Estraderm (skin patch)	natural oestrogen	"
Harmogen (tablets)	synthetic oestrogen	"

hormones that are doing it—her belief is just as effective! If you can generate a similar level of belief in yourself and the innate ability of your mind to suppress unpleasant menopausal symptoms, you can achieve the same effect in a much more satisfying way.

Mental control over menopausal symptoms can be taught. Women can learn to imagine that their hands are getting hot or cold, and can actually control their temperature. When they use this technique to cool themselves down just as they feel a flush coming on, they are able to abort the flush. Biofeedback can also help (clinical psychologists often have the necessary equipment) but it is theoretically possible to train yourself without any equipment at all. Try it—practise imagining that your hands are getting very hot and that they are the route by which you can lose the excess heat from your body. If you succeed, you will have fewer flushes and the ones you have will be less severe.

Why bother, you may ask, when you can simply take HRT? The reason is that HRT is not as satisfactory an answer as you might think from hearing effusions such as those from Ms O'Mara. First of all, progestogens can have side-effects such as bloating, weight gain, breast swelling and tenderness. They may depress your mood. They may make you feel thoroughly pre-menstrual ... and then they induce the nuisance of bleeding. And you thought that was all over with!

If you suffer from diabetes, migraine, fibroids, endometriosis, hypertension, hyperlipidaemia, epilepsy or liver problems, you should not take HRT. It could make your condition worse. If you're at high risk of breast cancer you should not take HRT; it is likely to increase the risk. This warning particularly applies to those who've already had breast disease, but women to whom two or more of the following risk factors apply would be wise to avoid adding further to their personal risk by using HRT: close relatives (sisters, mother, aunts) who've had breast cancer; periods starting before the age of 12; use of oral contraceptives starting in teens, continued use of oral contraceptives for five years or more; no full-term pregnancies; obesity.

The big question-mark hovering over HRT concerns its potential for increasing cancer risks. We know that oestrogen alone significantly increases endometrial cancers, which is why it should only be used by women who've had hysterectomies; but can the combined preparations in use today also increase cancer? This is evidence to suggest that there is 50 per cent excess risk of breast cancer risk when HRT is used for more than 10 years—a rise that corresponds with the increase in breast cancer with delayed menopause. But—and this is the worry—it may be too early to judge precisely how cancer risks change with HRT. Cancer is a disease with a long latency period; it can develop decades after contact with the cancer-causing substance. And modern types of HRT have not been used for long enough for anyone to be sure of the size of any possible excess risk.

The cancers that are most likely to increase with hormone treatment of any sort are those of sex-hormone sensitive tissues: the breasts, womb, ovaries, vagina. With rare cancers, it's relatively easy for medical statisticians to detect an increase, but it's much more difficult to tell when a drug causes a rise in a common cancer. Unfortunately, cancer of the breast is very common in post-menopausal women. There has been a steady rise in breast cancer mortality over recent decades and we would be foolhardy to presume that some, at least, of this rise is not due to our increased exposure to sex hormones from a wide range of sources.

While even a slight increase of breast cancer risk could mean thousands of extra deaths, defenders of HRT would point out that deaths linked with osteoporosis are reduced, and in some studies, deaths from all causes are lower in women who take HRT. One is bound to ask, however, whether this effect is due to the greater affluence of such women; HRT is still something of a middle-class treatment and by far the strongest predictors of longevity are money and privileged social class.

The medical establishment's strongest argument in favour of HRT is its ability to protect women from osteoporosis. This begs many questions. In particular, it ignores the fact that lifestyle changes will also provide such protection, and promote general health in the safest possible way. Osteoporosis is a lifestyle problem and the lifestyles that cause it also cause most of the other types of illness to which the people of Western industrialized nations are prone.

But in order to confront this problem, we must also confront the realities of life and health in today's Britain. Successive governments have demonstrated their preference for letting women take drugs for avoidable illness, rather than ensuring that everyone can afford sufficient fresh fruit and vegetables to meet their nutritional needs. Cigarette smoking is another major risk factor for osteoporosis, but how many women—or doctors—are aware of this? In view of the strength of the tobacco industry, and the large contribution from cigarette tax to government revenue, maybe we should not be surprised at the general level of ignorance. Let them have HRT—on the NHS—seems to go the argument.

If you use HRT to avoid osteoporosis, you have to continue taking it for the rest of your life. When women stop taking it, there's a rebound period of very rapid bone loss when their bones quickly shed all the tissue that was artificially sustained by the hormones. This then is a short-sighted solution to the problem—especially in view of the unknown long term risks.

This is not to say that all use of HRT is irrational. Women who have had hysterectomies and who are suffering severe menopausal symptoms as a consequence, benefit markedly from HRT. I believe it makes sense to cushion the effects of surgical hormone disruption in this way. And such women can safely take oestrogen alone, thus avoiding the unpleasant effects of progestogens. HRT may make sense for women who, despite their efforts to eat well and exercise, are still greatly troubled by night sweats and unable to get the rest they need. And it may make sense as an interim measure for women who are working on re-balancing their lives and their bodies, but who have had such severely unbalanced hormones—perhaps because of food sensitivity or illness—that the transition to good health is slow. We should not sacrifice quality of life for an exaggerated fear of what seems, overall, to be a reasonably safe type of therapy.

My research has convinced me, however, that to use HRT as a substitute for a healthy lifestyle is foolish and foolhardy. Personally, I know it's not for me: I'm in the high-risk group for breast cancer—my sister died of it—and I'm not going to take anything that could increase that risk.

Stopping HRT should be a gradual process. If you're taking it now, try reducing the dose slowly to see if you can manage without. If you suffer severe symptoms after a month without the tablets, return to using them for six months then try stopping again. Most women are perfectly well off without it when they're over the first couple of years of the menopause.

For those women who have not yet reached menopause, the way to avoid the miseries of a chaotic hormone shift is to prepare for it well in advance. You can't start changing your lifestyle too soon. Build up your bones with plenty of good food and exercise and by giving up cigarettes well before the menopause, when your hormones will support continued bone growth; those whose bones are strong in the first place are not likely to develop osteoporosis. Sort out your PMT problems by following the advice in this book so that you're less susceptible to menopausal distress when your periods begin to tail off. And junk your apprehensions about the menopause: by looking after yourself well, you'll stay well, retain your looks, and you'll sail through the change.

Menopause need not be a problem. Make sure it won't be your problem: it's your choice.

CHAPTER ELEVEN

Avoiding Hysterectomy

Hysterectomy is the most common major surgical operation for women. One in five women in Britain have had a hysterectomy by the age of 75; around 80,000 of these operations are performed every year and the rate is rising steadily. Hysterectomy is very closely tied in with hormone problems, both because long-standing imbalances cause the symptoms that make it necessary, and because the operation itself frequently leads to hormone deficiencies.

There are several types of hysterectomy and the particular operation a woman has depends partly on the reasons for it and partly on her surgeon's preferences. Hysterectomy means removal of the uterus, and, usually, the fallopian tubes attached to it. A total hysterectomy includes removal of the cervix, while subtotal or partial hysterectomy involves amputation of the uterus above the cervix. Oöphorectomy means removal of an ovary; bilateral oöphorectomy is removal of both ovaries. Salpingo-oöphorectomy is removal of both ovaries and fallopian tubes.

The operation can be done through the abdominal wall, with a vertical cut down from the navel or a horizontal cut near the hairline (the 'bikini cut'); this is usually preferable because it seems to heal better and the scar is less obvious. Alternatively, surgeons can do a vaginal hysterectomy, where the uterus is removed through the vagina without cutting into the abdomen. This is more difficult for the surgeon to do well, but it usually heals faster.

Hysterectomy is major surgery however it's carried out. It requires a general anaesthetic and about 10 days in hospital. Most women recover sufficiently to return to their normal lives within about two months but plenty of rest is needed after the operation. Although you'll be getting around after a week or so, even housework will be too much for the first month of convalescence. Most women feel it's a year before they're completely well.

Hysterectomy can be a life-saving operation. If you have cancer of the uterus (endometrial cancer), invasive cervical cancer, or cancer of the ovaries, it is usually the only answer. About 10 per cent of hysterectomies are for cancer. Other reasons are heavy, painful periods, chronic abdominal pain and pain with intercourse; possible causes include fibroids, endometriosis, prolapse, and pelvic infection. Problems of childbirth—a ruptured or inverted uterus, or massive uncontrollable haemorrhage—although rare, can also require immediate hysterectomy.

In an Oxford study of pre-menopausal women, the most common reasons for hysterectomy were abnormal bleeding (38 per cent), fibroids (37 per cent), prolapse (6 per cent), endometriosis (6 per cent) and cancer (5 per cent). The reasons for abnormal bleeding are rarely found; in most of these cases, the organs the surgeon removes seem completely normal.

Fibroids, benign growths in or attached to the uterus, are very common but often cause no symptoms. About 30 per cent of women have fibroids but they may be quite small. If they grow large or they're in such a position that they press on sensitive structures in the abdomen, they have to be removed. Many surgeons will do a hysterectomy under these circumstances, although, as I shall explain later, this is rarely the only option.

Endometriosis is a condition where hormone-sensitive cells from the uterine lining grow in the abdomen, often on the outside of the uterus, where they swell and bleed with each menstrual cycle. This causes pain and heavy periods.

Prolapse means misplacement of the uterus (or other organs such as the bladder). The uterus can fall into the wrong position in the abdomen when the ligaments which hold it in place get stretched, and this lead to pain and bleeding. Sometimes, the uterus can fall into the vagina. This can happen in older women whose tissues have lost their strength and elasticity so that they no longer support the uterus.

Pelvic infection (pelvic inflammatory disease, or PID) can follow childbirth; it can also occur as a result of sexually transmitted infections including chlamydia, gonorrhoea, and nonspecific urethritis (NSU), or sterilization. PID has become much more common in recent years with increased sexual freedom and the use of IUDs (the coil, or intra-uterine device). An IUD containing copper can set up a chronic inflammation in the uterus and its copper content interferes with immunity, making you particularly susceptible to PID. In addition, some doctors believe that infection travels up the string on the IUD through the cervix. Usually, removal of the IUD (don't ever be persuaded to have another if you've had PID!), and antibiotics will be sufficient to clear the infection, although it may be years before you're completely free of pain. If the condition becomes chronic, a hysterectomy may be recommended.

There's a lot of evidence to suggest that, in the United States, the majority of hysterectomies carried out are unnecessary, but the situation is less clear-cut in Britain where doctors don't make money from extra surgery and NHS resources are chronically stretched. Nevertheless, it's likely that even here, many women undergo hysterectomy when they need not; in Norway, where women live longer than in the UK, hysterectomy rates are half what they are here. In the rapidly expanding private sector of British medicine, where surgery is highly profitable, hysterectomy rates are rising particularly quickly.

Apart from economic incentives for expensive surgery in private hospitals, the main reasons for our rising hysterectomy rates are social and cultural. An increase in hormone problems caused by the way we live contributes to increasing gynaecological illness, and women may be less willing to put up with it than previously. Consultations for new cases of abnormal uterine bleeding went up by 73 per cent between 1971 and 1981 according to surveys carried out by the Royal College of General Practitioners.

Family doctors vary widely in their willingness to refer women for hysterectomy. Individual attitudes to women, gynaecological problems, and to surgery play a large part in determining how they respond to patients who consult them with problems like excessive pain or bleeding, problems which cannot be measured directly. Their judgement will be influenced by factors that may have nothing to do with the woman's condition. If your doctor sees you as a troublesome or difficult patient, he may refer you to a consultant simply to get rid of you. One GP, quoted in *Woman's Journal*, was quite candid: 'I became aware of being quite definitely unsympathetic when older women came in with the predictable list of complaints ... No wonder there are so many 'routine' hysterectomies—it is the easiest, quickest way of getting a patient off their hands and out of your surgery.'

Some doctors' and surgeons' beliefs make them especially willing to propose hysterectomy. Many imagine that the operation does far less harm than in fact it does. Many believe that women who don't want babies, who are infertile for any reason, or past whatever the doctor thinks is the right age for having babies, don't need their wombs and are better off without them. Medicine is a male-dominated profession, where women's organs are little appreciated and women's concerns often dismissed as being neurotic and irrational. If the uterus were a male organ, we can be sure there would be far fewer hysterectomies!

A Swiss study adds weight to these suspicions. Male gynaecologists, it was found, did twice as many hysterectomies as their female colleagues. Regrettably, the majority of surgeons are male.

There have always been fervent (male) advocates of hysterectomy: in the late sixties, one American gynaecologist wrote that when the uterus is no longer required for pregnancy, it becomes 'a useless, bleeding, symptom-producing, potentially cancer-bearing organ, and therefore should be removed'. He was far from being alone in holding this view. An article in the medical journal *Patient Care* in 1980 asserted that: 'The uterus can be a tremendous nuisance after it has finished its childbearing function. If a woman is willing to withstand the nuisance, well and good; let her keep her uterus. But if she wants freedom from its problems, her wish should be honoured.' And in Britain, similar attitudes are widespread. Estelle Gunstock was 44 when a benign ovarian cyst was diagnosed. The surgeon decided that the ovary should be removed and asked her how old she was. On learning she'd reached the ripe old age of 44, he decided to remove the uterus at the same time!

The ovaries, too, are considered potentially hazardous and 'unnecessary' for older women. Many American doctors are taught that the ovaries should always be removed during hysterectomy in a woman over 40.

So if you are told you need a hysterectomy, always make sure you're well informed about all the options. If your problem is bleeding or pain, you may be able to cure it without surgery. If surgery is unavoidable, make sure you're not going to lose any more organs than is strictly necessary. Don't let those assumptions about their nuisance value lead a surgeon to remove more than he need.

Beliefs about the nuisance value of internal sexual organs are not restricted to male gynaecologists, of course. Many women, tired of years of pain, messy periods, and contraceptive bother, are only too ready to have their wombs removed. My friend Jo just wanted to get rid of the lot and worked hard to persuade her doctor to sanction the operation. When I had a lot of trouble with my periods, I used to imagine hysterectomy would be an attractive option. But while hysterectomy can be essential and can (once you've recovered from the operation) make you feel much better providing your gynaecological problems cannot be solved any other way, it isn't something to be contemplated lightly. It can cause serious physiological and psychological damage.

Studies of women who have had hysterectomies show that they suffer considerably more illness than women who have had other operations, or no surgery at all. These effects last for many years after the operation.

In the United States, medical sociologist Sonja McKinley asked 8,000 women between the ages of 45 and 55 about their health. 30 per cent of her sample had been hysterectomized. These women reported more chronic illness, used twice as many prescription medicines as the remaining 70 per cent of the sample, and were significantly more likely to describe their health as 'worse than that of others'. On the basis of her research, Dr McKinley believes that hysterectomy has far-reaching and dangerous effects on health.

Psychological problems are particularly common. After hysterectomy with oöphorectomy, women are four times as likely to suffer clinical depression; those who lose their uterus but retain their ovaries are three times as likely to get seriously depressed as other women of the same age. Women who have had psychiatric care before hysterectomy are 10 times as likely to need it after the operation. What's more, this particular type of mental illness is more difficult to treat and lasts longer.

Marital problems and divorce increase after hysterectomy. One factor that contributes to this problem is loss of sexual feeling and desire. It is commonly asserted by doctors that sexual feeling is unchanged by hysterectomy, presumably because of the widespread belief that the clitoris is the only sexually responsive genital organ; the evidence shows this to be untrue. For many women, orgasm involves the uterus and deep stimulation is necessary for sexual satisfaction; loss of the uterus and its associated structures means loss of a crucial orgasmic organ.

Loss of sexual feeling is far from inevitable. For some women, sex is better after hysterectomy than before, especially if intercourse had been painful or they were afraid of getting pregnant—though sterilization, a relatively minor operation, will solve that problem much more easily! It has been estimated, however, that between 33 and 46 per cent of women lose most of their sexual responsiveness.

This change may be related to the loss of their ovaries, even when they have not been surgically removed; recent evidence shows that the ovaries often die or diminish in function after removal of the uterus. The blood supply to the ovaries is provided mainly by the uterine artery, which comes directly from the uterus. During hysterectomy, this artery is cut off and sealed so there is no longer sufficient blood to sustain healthy ovaries, which shrivel and die. This leads to predictable loss of hormone production.

Even when the ovaries manage to survive, loss of the uterus leads to hormone distruption. The uterus itself produces prostaglandins and hormone-like substances which contribute to the feedback systems that maintain hormone balance. The ovaries may require cyclical changes in the uterus in order to function as they should. Hysterectomy often causes hormone-related problems like hot flushes and weepiness within a day or so of surgery; severe menopausal symptoms develop in 50 per cent of women who have a hysterectomy even when an ovary is left intact and every woman who loses her ovaries will suffer a sudden and drastic menopause.

In her book *No More Hysterectomies* (Thorsons), gynaecologist Dr Vicki Hufnagel lists the following symptoms that occur as a result of the loss of ovarian function: osteoporosis, arthritis, cardiovascular disease, hot flushes, insomnia, depression, loss of sexual desire, masculinization, chronic migraines, bowel dysfunction, generalized fatigue, neurological complaints, increased allergies, loss of normal body fat distribution, loss of orgasm, severe PMT, rapid aging of the skin, bloating, cyclic oedema, obesity, thyroid dysfunction, memory loss, loss of sex drive.

The complications of the operation itself can add to women's problems. The death rate due to hysterectomy is between one and two per thousand; but for every woman who dies, many more become seriously ill. General anaesthesia is not without risk; brain damage and liver disease are just two of the adverse reactions it can produce. Infection develops after about a third of abdominal hysterectomies; it's less of a problem after vaginal hysterectomy but this, as we shall see, can cause other illness. Peritonitis and pelvic abcesses can develop months after the operation.

A Canadian study found that 4 per cent of the complications of hysterectomy required re-admission to hospital within two years for further surgery. This can be because of adhesions—scar tissue within the abdomen which can wrap around the ovaries, making them massive and painful. Adhesions can lead to the bowel, fallopian tubes or other organs sticking to the remains of the uterus or to each other; it can cause obstructions in the bowel or twists that trap the faeces so that the bowel no longer works as it should.

Damage to the nerves or to the urinary organs can cause further problems. Sometimes a ureter (one of the tubes leading from the bladder) gets cut during surgery so that urine leaks into the abdomen; nerves are often cut, causing leg pain, weakness and numbness in more than 10 per cent of women. Urinary tract complications, including infections, affect a further 10 per cent.

The loss of supporting structures within the abdomen can lead to yet more problems. Vaginal hysterectomy, which involves pulling the uterus away from the organs which surround it, can destroy the internal organization so that the pelvic organs collapse inside. Prolapse can occur up to 10 years later.

Finally, blood vessel damage can cause thrombosis and internal bleeding, while hormonal change increases the risk of all types of cardiovascular problems. The risk of heart disease is trebled for women who have hysterectomies before the natural menopause.

Obviously, if there's any alternative to hysterectomy, you would be wise to take it. Alternatives often do exist, some medical, some surgical; and lifestyle change to rebalance hormones could solve the problems that led you or your doctor to contemplate this drastic operation. You're playing for high stakes; it's worth taking time and spending money where necessary to cure your condition without losing your uterus.

Fibroids, endometriosis, and heavy or painful periods are the most common reasons for hysterectomy. All these are hormone-related problems. Most doctors will try to control them with drugs before suggesting hysterectomy, but if you fail to deal with the lifestyle problems that cause hormone imbalance, you'll be fighting a losing battle.

Your health must be your number one priority. It'll take time to get everything right, but if you're forced to have a hysterectomy that will take a lot of time and pleasure out of your life too. Change your diet to make sure you eat as chapters four and five suggest. If you've been dieting to lose weight, STOP NOW! Eat well, but eat right. Fat women are malnourished—not over-nourished. Use nutritional supplements, particularly essential fatty acids, vitamins A, B$_6$ and folic acid, and magnesium, zinc, and iron if you have bleeding problems. Contact the Women's Nutritional Advisory Centre (page 166) for individual diet recommendations. Step up your activity levels; find activities that suit you and do them regularly and frequently. Sort out stresses in your life that will tend to add to hormone imbalance; counselling, meditation and a lot of hard thinking will all help. Attend to allergies by seeking out allergen sources and eliminating them from your life. Give up smoking.

Complementary therapies such as acupuncture, herbalism and homoeopathy may help your body to achieve a better balance. Look for a therapist with whom you feel comfortable and whom you trust, and who has been through a thorough training in his or her discipline. See 'Helpful organizations' (page 165) for addresses of centres and for information on therapies.

If all these changes don't solve the problem, at least they will make you fitter for any operation. You'll suffer less if you're as healthy as possible when you go in for surgery.

Drug therapy may be capable of reversing pathological changes, and it's likely to be more effective if you're getting all the nutrients you need. Having studied the question of prescription drugs in great detail, both in my research in medical sociology and for the books I've co-written, including *Cured to Death; the effects of prescription drugs* (Secker and Warburg), I believe that they can have a useful role when safer options have been tried and prove insufficient. So while I have great reservations about the use of medical hormone therapies, I think they have a place and should be tried before hysterectomy.

Danazol (Danol), which is an analogue (chemical copy) of a male sex hormone which suppresses oestrogen and increases testosterone levels, is one drug that may be offered if you have endometriosis. Try it if safer measures prove insufficient. You may also be offered progesterone in one of its various forms. Natural progesterone suppositories are safest but may not be sufficient to reverse your condition; see if you can at least try them first if your doctor considers progesterone therapy is necessary. Synthetic forms, including tablets and injected progesterones like Depoprovera, are more hazardous but they are still safer than hysterectomy.

Some surgical options are less drastic than hysterectomy but you may have to search to find a surgeon who is skilled in these operations. Endometriosis, ovarian cysts and fibroids can be removed by delicate surgery or, preferably, laser treatment, without loss of any major organs. Myomectomy is the technical term for removal of fibroids while leaving the uterus.

Prolapse and misplacement of the uterus can be surgically treated by re-suspension of the organs within the abdomen. This conservative treatment is less popular with many surgeons than hysterectomy, but if you insist that you really want to keep your uterus, it should be possible to find a surgeon who will respect your wishes.

Sometimes, there really is no choice about it. However unpleasant the prospect of surgery (and I'm not going to pretend it's not, in the too-cheerful manner of the reassurance merchants), you may have to face it. As I've said earlier, the operation can be life-saving.

I remember the occasion when my mother had a hysterectomy very well. For months she had been desperately weak and tired, she'd been lying on a sofa, pale and scarcely able to move. She looked very beautiful in her wine-coloured housecoat, like a Victorian heroine; but her life was bleeding away after five difficult births. Something drastic had to be done. The operation was a relief; she looked much more healthy afterwards and had more energy.

That was thirty years ago, when the support that's available now did not exist. My mother went through a very trying menopause for years after her operation. Today, you can get help with post-hysterectomy hormone imbalances; oestrogen replacement therapy—with added testosterone if you've lost your libido—makes sense if you suffer from severe menopausal symptoms after the operation. The risks are low and the benefits can be dramatic.

There's also a network of hysterectomy advice and support groups all over Britain. These are co-ordinated by Ann Webb, a health visitor who herself has had a hysterectomy; her address is 11 Henryson Road, Brockley, London SE4 1HL (telephone 081 690 5987).

By the time you're offered a hysterectomy, your problems may be far advanced and alternative options may not be sufficient. The best answer is to take action early, when safe options still exist. Most of the problems that lead to hysterectomy are caused by severe hormone imbalance, and action to ensure the best possible balance at all times will make it very unlikely that you'll ever be in the position of having to contemplate hysterectomy.

When I was getting a lot of pain five years ago, my GP diagnosed fibroids. He was able to feel them by bimanual examination, using both hands to investigate my uterus and associated organs. He laughed, saying it was my age; I knew him well enough to understand the joke and I laughed too. Nevertheless I was naturally concerned; I knew nothing about fibroids.

'What happens next?' I wanted to know.

'Well,' he said, 'You might be offered a hysterectomy. It's difficult to remove fibroids and most surgeons are unwilling to do it.'

'Would you go for that, if you were a woman?'

'No.' He was suddenly serious. 'I'd grit my teeth and hang on for as long as I possibly could. Meantime, you could try evening primrose oil.'

I began to search for information about fibroids and soon realized that my pre-menstrual symptoms were part of the same problem. My hormones were out of balance. So I began to read about the problem and slowly pieced together the strategy for re-balancing that I've been describing in this book. I no longer have pain, and no longer have any sign of fibroids. I would say that fibroids are not progressive providing you get the balance of your hormones right; they can shrink and cease to produce symptoms.

I was lucky in that my fibroids were identified early and I was able to find out about appropriate natural treatment; my doctor's suggestion about evening primrose oil had been spot-on, though that was just the beginning. But if I'd dealt with my PMT earlier, those fibroids would probably never had developed. And that's the real message of this book: that we can and must solve our hormone imbalance problems while natural remedies can still be used.

I have (so far!) avoided hysterectomy. I believe that the strategy I began to adopt when the possibility of hysterectomy was first raised has tremendously reduced the chances that I'll ever have to undergo this (or any other) operation. At the same time, I know that my actions will reduce my risk of having breast cancer, ovarian cancer, menopausal problems and osteoporosis. When I start to get sloppy about my diet and lifestyle, I remind myself of these benefits. Natural health is far better than anything medicine or surgery can create!

CHAPTER TWELVE
A Balanced Life for Today's Woman

As I hope the previous chapters have illustrated, I believe hormone problems can be solved by the adoption of the right lifestyle. Our hormone balance is a product of the way we live; if we fail to provide for our personal needs, hormone-related problems result. Imbalance, leading to symptoms ranging from PMT through infertility to osteoporosis, is very common indeed, a reflection of the general lack of concern with human needs in a world where health is subordinated to economic profit.

In this book, I have described the requirements for hormone health: a varied diet of wholesome, nutritious food; a level of everyday activity that matches the capabilities of our bodies; avoidance of pollutants that can interfere with the creation of hormones and their metabolism, and acceptance of our feminine nature, different in its needs and strengths from that of the male.

Women run into hormone problems because the provisions of the modern world often ignore our fundamental needs. We are encouraged to eat food that doesn't provide the nutrients on which we depend, because processed, denatured food is more profitable for the business interests that control it. We are encouraged to be sedentary because cars, labour saving machines and packaged entertainment make money, while jobs keep us static in a technological world. We are encouraged to be passive, accepting, unquestioning, because we cause less trouble if we just fit in with the dominant order.

But our hormone balance is inherently delicate, readily thrown out of harmony. In an ideal world, our needs and the demands of our culture would not be in conflict; but our world is less than ideal. Conflicts exist on every level, often unrecognized and sometimes apparently irreconcilable.

The fundamental requirements of hormone health are the basic requirements of general health for everyone. The imbalance in women's hormone systems is just one sign of damage. Men suffer a different pattern of illness; they are more likely to develop heart disease, a modern epidemic against which female hormones provide some protection. Our peculiarly female problems may seem trivial in a male-dominated world, but for many women, they can be incapacitating.

Whatever health problem we like to consider, the same issues come up again and again: diet, exercise, pollution, our attitudes to ourselves. When we act to solve these problems for ourselves to achieve a better hormone balance, we are taking action on fronts that should concern everyone.

Hormone health isn't just a physical problem—few aspects of health are—it's also a cultural issue. Culture is a product of combined human consciousness, the sum of our beliefs, attitudes, thought, and creativity. It determines how we cope with the world, how we react to everything that happens to us; it determines our relationships and the way we think. Our culture is dominated by male assumptions, male priorities; technology and economics, the priorities of business, have created a world ecological crisis which can only be met with a resurgence of feminine values.

In this patriarchal culture, women have become passive adjuncts to male-dominated institutions. Feminine values are concerned with caring; women put lives first—the lives of children, families and communities. But our intuitive knowledge that these are the things that really matter has become submerged under the imperatives of a materialist culture that makes little provision for social and emotional relationships.

Being female means having to fit caring—for ourselves and our families—around the demands of economic survival. Women rightly refuse to relinquish their deeper responsibilities but the effect is that being female means being regarded as a second-class, unreliable citizen. Women carry a double load of responsibility, looking after homes and families as well as juggling jobs. We work longer hours for less reward than men, because much of our work is unpaid, underpaid, and undervalued. With all these demands, it's crucial that we maintain our health; yet because of them, it's difficult to find the time and energy to look after ourselves and our children properly.

Recognizing the inequalities in society, some women seek to

emulate men, rejecting their own female nature. And while they may protect themselves from some of the worst forms of exploitation, they too pay a price, for our sexual nature is undeniable and its manifestations impinge all the more painfully on our consciousness when we try to deny them. If we dislike our femininity because of its implications, we will suffer, rather than enjoy, the effects of this femininity. It's difficult to accept ourselves fully as women if being female, to us, means being inferior.

As we feel, so we become. The masculinized woman, competing in the business world with its male priorities, actually begins to produce more male hormones. Women who take on the male ethic of the power struggle become susceptible to heart disease like men. The padding in the shoulders of the power-dresser is a cultural reflection of physiological adaptation. Equally, the home-body who devotes her life to her family in an exaggerated 'feminine' role also suffers the distortion of her nature. Femininity, with its cultural connotations of passivity, self-denial and obsession with youth, fertility and prettiness, can bring real suffering when women are no longer capable of bearing children.

We have to achieve a balance throughout our lives. Balance in our lifestyles to support the physiological balance of our bodies, and balance in our attitudes so that we can appreciate and enjoy our femininity without becoming obsessed with our ability to produce babies. We have to balance our social needs, and those of our dependents, with our personal needs; to balance the needs of our families against the well-being of the planet.

As women, we are uniquely equipped to juggle all these issues, for we live all our lives in a changing balance which is sensitive to everything that happens to us. We can recognize the importance of the felt, the unknown; for in our own lives these are phenomena that directly affect us. We understand flux and change in a fundamental way because we are constantly changing as our hormone balance shifts in the cycles of fertility. But most urgently, we need to learn to appreciate these feminine qualities, to value ourselves and our nature sufficiently to change the culture that we help to create.

Feminine nature, with its cyclical hormonal changes, is intimately connected with the cycles of birth, life and death. Masculine nature, which dominates our culture, is more linear in its quality. The survival of our planet depends on a new understanding of cyclical processes, for these are sustainable in the long term as linear processes are not. Women have a responsibility to assert the importance of the cyclical paradigm which is built into their own bodies, to emphasize their way of being in the wider world context. Linear thinking is the paradigm of the economic models that predominate today; until we adopt cyclical models, the destruction of natural processes which so threatens our future will continue.

Women are starting to fight back against the anti-life ethos that allows people and other animals to be sacrificed to corporate greed; but we do not always recognize how ecological issues affect us directly, nor how our actions contribute to them. In working towards our personal balance, we can help to create a better balance in the world.

The forces that damage women's hormone health also damage the whole balance of life on earth. The production of contaminated food which lacks nutritional value turns our fields into green deserts where virtually all life except the farmer's cash crop has been exterminated. The creation of synthetic chemicals, pesticides and additives that disrupt our metabolic systems produces waste that poisons the air, rivers and seas. The ubiquitous motor cars and machines that lure us into allowing our muscles to waste away, pollute the air and add to the greenhouse effect that harms the planet.

We are dependent on the integrity of the fragile mantle of life on earth just as surely as a baby depends on the placenta. Only through ecological balance can the world provide good food, break down our wastes, and maintain the purity of air and water so that we can survive. Our demand for natural health is at the forefront of the struggle for a way of living that will make life sustainable indefinitely.

Natural health does not depend on male-dominated institutions like the medical profession or the drug companies; it works at a personal level, with changes in the ways we act and think. The feminine approach is non-violent; it avoids surgical and medical violence to our bodies in the context of a caring society. This new way of living is part of a larger movement towards a new balance between the sexes, between individuals and society, between humankind and the natural world.

I look forward to a future where caring counts; a future where sympathy is no longer dismissed as sentimentality and feminine intuition doesn't get swamped under hard 'facts' selected to fit exploitative masculine values. Our history of male dominance has led us to rely on others, on experts and institutions, and to ignore the fact that one half of our brain operates under female principles. Women must become more responsible, more self-reliant, the prime movers in the new direction of our culture so that our nurturing prerogatives can flower to create a world where all life can thrive.

Helpful organizations

If you write to any of the following organizations, always send a stamped addressed envelope with your enquiry.

British Acupuncture Register and Directory
34 Alderney Street
London SW1 4VE
071 834 1012

British Pregnancy Advisory Service
Austy Manor, Wootton Wawen
Solihull
West Midlands B95 6BX
05642 3225
(Offer sterilization and abortion services.)

The Council for Acupuncture
Suite 1
19a Cavendish Square
London W1M 9AD
071 409 1440

Foresight
The Association for the Promotion of Pre-Conceptual Care
The Old Vicarage
Church Lane
Witley, Godalming
Surrey GU8 5PN
042879 4500.
(Advises women with infertility problems and those who want to maximize their chances of having a healthy baby.)

Friends of the Earth
377 City Road
London EC1V 1NA
071 837 0731

The Soil Association
86 Colston Street
Bristol BS1 5BB
0272 290661
(Information on organic food and farming.)

Women's Health & Reproductive Rights Information Centre (WHRRIC),
52 Featherstone Street
London EC1 8RT
071 251 6332
(Information on women's health issues.)

Women and Medical Practice (WAMP)
666 High Road
Tottenham, London N17
081 885 2277
(Offers counselling and information to women on medical and health questions.)

Women's Nutritional Advisory Service and Pre-menstrual Ten-

sion Advisory Service
PO Box 268
Hove, East Sussex BN3 6RH
0273 771366
(Personalized diet and lifestyle
plans for optimum health and
general advice on nutrition for
women.)

USA
National   Health   Information
Center
PO Box 1133,
Washington,
DC (800 336 4797 outside MD)

National Women's Network
244 7th Street SE,
Washington,
DC 20003

North   American   Menopause
Society
NY Academy of Sciences,
2E 63rd Street,
New York,
NY 10021

Premenstrual Syndrome Access
PO Box 9326, Madison,
WI 53715
(800 237 4666)

Women's Association for Research in Menopause
128 E. 56th St,
New York,
NY 10022

Women's Health Advisory Service
PO Box 31000,
Phoenix,
AZ 85046

Women's   Health   Information
Center (US)
Boston Women's Health Book
Collective,
47 Nichols Ave., Watertown,
MA 02172

Canada
Health & Welfare Canada,
National Day Care Information
Centre,
Tunney's Pasture,
Ottawa,
Ontario K1A 1B5

National Council of Women of
Canada
270 MacLaren St, Room 20,
Ottawa,
Ontario K2P 0M3
(613) 233-4953

Women's   Health   Education
Network
PO Box 1276,
Truro, Nova Scotia
B2N 5N2

Women's Research Centre
301–2515 Burrard St,
Vancouver, British Columbia
V6J 3T6

Australia
Australian Institute of Health
Bennett House,
Hospital Point, Acton,
ACT GPO Box 570,
ACT 2601
(062) 43 5000

Menopause   Clinic   (Royal
Hospital for Women)
188 Oxford Street,
Paddington
2021 (339 4111)

Women's Health Care Association
Inc.
92 Thomas St,
W. Perth,
WA 6005
(09) 321 2833

Women's Health Advisory Service
PO Box 1096,
Bankstown 2200
(708 4794)

Women's Information Switch-
board
122 Kintore Ave., Adelaide,
SA 5000
(08) 223 2833

Women's Medical Centre
8th Floor, Challis House,
10 Martin Place,
Sydney
2000 (231 2366)

New Zealand
Department of Health
PO Box 5013,
Wellington

National Council of Women of
New Zealand (Inc)
PO Box 12117,
Wellington North

New Zealand Federation of
Fitness Centres Inc.
PO Box 44029,
Auckland

Nutrition Society of New Zealand
Inc.
Dept. of Food Technology,
Massey University,
Palmerston North

Recommended reading

Gear, Alan: *The New Organic Food Guide* (Dent).

Grant, Doris and Joice, Jean: *Food Combining for Health* (Thorsons).

Grant, Ellen: *The Bitter Pill: How Safe is the 'Perfect Contraceptive'?* (Elm Tree Books).

Kenton, Leslie & Susannah: *Raw Energy* (Century).

Kitzinger, Sheila: *Women as Mothers* (Fontana).

Mansfield, Peter and Monro, Jean: *Chemical Children: How to Protect Your Family from Harmful Pollutants* (Century).

Melville, Arabella and Johnson, Colin: *Alternatives to Drugs* (Fontana); *Eat Yourself Thin* (Michael Joseph).

Robertson, James: *The Sane Alternative: a Choice of Futures* Available from James Robertson, The Old Bakehouse, Cholsey, nr Wallingford, Oxon OX10 9NU.

Stewart, Maryon: *Beat PMT Through Diet* (Ebury Press).

Stoppard, Miriam: *The Pregnancy and Birth Book* (Dorling Kindersley).

Westcott, Patsy: *Alternative Health Care for Women* (Grapevine).

References

Abraham, Guy. Nutritional factors in the etiology of the premenstrual tension syndromes. *Journal of Reproductive Medicine*, 28 (7), 1983, 446–461.

Atik, S.O. Zinc and senile osteoporosis. *J. Amer. Geriatrics Soc.*, 31, 12, 1983, 790–1.

Biskind, M. Inactivation of testosterone proprionate in the liver following vitamin B complex deficiency: alteration of the estrogen-androgen equilibrium. *Endocrinology*, 32, 1975, 97–102.

Bland, Jeffrey (Ed.) *Medical Applications of Clinical Nutrition*. New Canaan: Keats, 1983.

Boston Women's Health Book Collective. *The New Our Bodies, Ourselves*. Penguin. 1989.

Bonen, A. Exercise-related disturbances in the menstrual cycle. In Borer, K.T. et al. (eds), *Frontiers of Exercise Biology*. Champaign, Ill.: Human Kinetics Publishers Inc., 1983.

British Medical Association and the Royal Pharmaceutical Society of Great Britain. *British National Formulary No. 17*. London: The Pharmaceutical Press, 1989.

Brush, Michael. *Understanding Premenstrual Tension*. London: Pan, 1984.

Bryce-Smith, D. Boron: a candidate for essentiality. *Felmore Health Publications, no. 151*.

Coulter, A. et al. Do British women undergo too many or too few hysterectomies? *Social Science and Medicine*, 27, 9, 1988, 987–994.

Dalton, Katharina. *Once a Month*. London: Fontana, 1978.

Davies, S. and Stewart, A. *Nutritional Medicine*. Pan Books, 1987.

Ehenreich, B. and English, D. *For Her Own Good: 150 years of the experts' advice to women*. London: Pluto, 1979.

Fioretti, Piero et al. *Postmenopausal Hormonal Therapy: Benefits and Risks*. New York: Raven Press, 1987.

Forbes, G. B. *Human Body Composition*. New York: Springer-Verlag, 1987.

Frisch, Rose. Exercise, Nutrition, Puberty and Fertility: delayed menarche and amenorrhoea. In Borer, K.T. et al. (eds), *Frontiers of Exercise Biology*. Champaign, Ill.: Human Kinetics Publishers Inc., 1983.

Gear, Alan. *The New Organic Food Guide*. London: Dent, 1987.

Grant, Doris and Joice, Jean. *Food Combining for Health* Wellingborough: Thorsons, 1984.

Grant, Ellen. *The Bitter Pill: How Safe is the 'Perfect Contraceptive'?* London: Elm Tree Books, 1985.

Hamburg, D. A. et al. Studies of distress in the menstrual cycle and the postpartum period. In: Michael, R.P. (ed.) *Endocrinology and Human Behaviour*. London: Oxford University Press, 1968.

Henderson, B.E. et al., Re-evaluating the role of progestogen therapy after the menopause. *Fertility and Sterility*, 49, 5, 1988, 9S–15S.

Hill, E.G. et al., Intensification of essential fatty acid deficiency in the rat by dietary trans fatty acids. *Journal of Nutrition*, 109, 1979, 1579.

"Hormone replacement therapy around and after the menopause: when and how?" *Drug and Therapeutics Bulletin*, 25, 9, 5 May 1987.

Hufnagel, Vicki. *No More Hysterectomies*. Thorsons, 1990.

Hunt, Kate and Vessey, Martin. Long-term effects of postmenopausal hormone therapy. *British Journal of Hospital Medicine*, 38 (5), 1987, 450–458.

Jansen, P.O. et al. The aging ovary. *Acta Obstet. Gynecol. Scand.* 106, 1982, 7–9.

Jones, D.Y. et al. Influence of dietary fat on menstrual cycle and menses length. *Human Nutrition and Clinical Nutrition*, 41 (5), 1987, 341–5.

Key, T.J.A. and Pike, M.C. The role of oestrogens and progestagens in the epidemiology and prevention of breast cancer. *British Journal of Cancer and Clinical Oncology*, 21, 1, 1988, 29–43.

Kitzinger, Sheila. *Women as Mothers*. London: Fontana, 1978.

Logue, C.M. and Moos, R.H. Positive perimenstrual changes: toward a new perspective on the menstrual cycle. *Journal of Psychosomatic Research*, 32, 1, 1988, 31–40.

McArdle, W.D. et al. *Exercise Physiology: Energy, Nutrition and Human Performance*. Philadelphia: Lea & Febinger, 1981.

Mastrovanni, L. and Paulsen, C. (eds.) *Aging, Reproduction and the Climacteric*. New York: Plenum, 1986.

Melville, Arabella and Johnson, Colin. *Cured to Death: the Effects of Prescription Drugs*. London: Secker & Warburg, 1982.

Melville, Arabella and Johnson, Colin. *Eat Yourself Thin*. London: Michael Joseph, 1990.

Mutrie, N. The psychological effects of exercise for women. In Borer, K.T. et al. (eds), *Frontiers of Exercise Biology*. Champaign, Ill.: Human Kinetics Publishers Inc., 1983.

Nielsen, F.H. et al. Effect of dietary boron on mineral, estrogen, and testosterone metabolism in postmenopausal women. *FASEB Journal*, 1, 1987, 394–397.

Nygaard, E. & Hede, K. Physiological profiles of the male and the female. In Macleod, D. et al., *Exercise: Benefits, Limits and Adaptations*. London: E. & F.N. Spon, 1987.

"Osteoporosis: prevention and treatment". *Drug and Therapeutics Bulletin*, 27, 1, 9 January 1989.

Passwater, Richard and Cranton, Elmer. *Trace Elements, Hair Analysis and Nutrition*. New Canaan: Keats, 1983.

Paul, A.A. and Southgate, D.A.T. *McCance and Widdowson's The Composition of Foods* (4th Edn.) London: HMSO, 1978.

Prior, J.C. Exercise-related adaptive changes of the menstrual cycle. In: McLeod, D. et al. (eds.) *Exercise: Benefits, Limits and Adaptations*. London: E & F.N. Spon, 1987.

Reitz, Rosetta. *Menopause: A Positive Approach*. London: Unwin, 1985.

Robertson, James: *The Sane Alternative: a Choice of Futures*. From Schumacher Society Book Service, 1983.

Rubinow, D.R. et al. Changes in plasma hormones across the menstrual cycle in patients with menstrually related mood disorder and in control subjects. *American Journal of Obstetrics and Gynecology*, 158, 1988, 5–11.

Scambler, A. and G. Menstrual symptoms, attitudes and consulting behaviour. *Social Science and Medicine*, 20, 10, 1985, 1065–1068.

Snowden, R. and Christian, B. (eds) *Patterns and Perceptions of Menstruation: A WHO international collaborative study.* London: Croom Helm, 1983.

Stewart, Maryon. *Beat PMT Through Diet.* London: Ebury Press, 1987.

Stoppard, Miriam: *The Pregnancy and Birth Book.* London: Dorling Kindersley, 1989.

Studd, J.W.W. and Whitehead, M. (eds.) *The Menopause.* Oxford: Blackwell Scientific, 1988.

Toth, Bela and Erickson, James. Reversal of the toxicity of hydrazine analogues by pyridoxine hydrochloride. *Toxicology*, 7, 1977, 31–36.

Weideger, Paula. *Female Cycles.* London: The Women's Press, 1978.

Westcott, Patsy: *Alternative Health Care for Women.* Wellingborough: Thorsons, 1987.

"Women athletes fend off cancer". *New Scientist*, 18 February 1988, p.27.

Wynn, Margaret and Wynn, Arthur. *Prevention of Handicap and the Health of Women.* London: Routledge and Kegan Paul, 1979.

Index